Understanding Multiple Myeloma

Cristina Gasparetto, MD
Associate Professor of Medicine
Director Multiple Myeloma Program
Duke University Medical Center

Dharshan Sivaraj
Duke University

JONES & BARTLETT
LEARNING

World Headquarters
Jones & Bartlett Learning
5 Wall Street
Burlington, MA 01803
978-443-5000
info@jblearning.com
www.jblearning.com

Jones & Bartlett Learning books and products are available through most bookstores and online booksellers. To contact Jones & Bartlett Learning directly, call 800-832-0034, fax 978-443-8000, or visit our website, www.jblearning.com.

14982-1

Production Credits

VP of Product Management: David D. Cella
Director of Product Management: Amanda Martin
Product Manager: Teresa Reilly
Product Assistant: Anna-Maria Forger
Production Manager: Daniel Stone
Marketing Manager: Lindsay White

Media Development Editor: Shannon Sheehan
Rights & Media Specialist: Wes DeShano
Cover Design: Scott Moden
Cover Image: © David Litman/Shutterstock
Composition: S4Carlisle Publishing Services
Printing and Binding: Edwards Brothers Malloy

ISBN: 978-1-284-14982-1

6048

Printed in the United States of America
22 21 20 19 18   10 9 8 7 6 5 4 3 2

Dedication

We dedicate this book to all our patients, caregivers and families who entrust us with their care. To our parents Alessandro & Gulia Gasparetto, Tham & Jega Sivaraj, as well as Alex Gasparetto Smith, we could not have published this book without your unconditional support in all aspects of our lives.

Contents

Preface

The purpose of this book is to provide a framework for patients, students, and health professionals alike to better understand the history, treatment, and behavior of the blood cancer multiple myeloma. We urge readers to make use of the footnotes and corresponding definitions located within each page for further clarity on multiple myeloma related terms. As a patient, becoming informed about the nature and treatment of this disease can help facilitate a more active and supportive relationship with the healthcare team. We hope that this book provides insight into where we have been, where we currently are, and where we are going, regarding our understanding of multiple myeloma.

Acknowledgments

We would like to extend our gratitude to the multiple myeloma team at Duke University, particularly Anderson Garrett, Jackie McIntyre, Deborah Russell, Kim Renee Nester, Emily Sellars, Indya Horton, Julia Hoyle, Ludmila Francescatto, Beth Mancuso, Scott Winkel, Therese Hennig, Angela Johns and Dr. Michael Green. Additionally, we would like to recognize the attending physicians of the Hematologic Malignancies and Cellular Therapy Division of the Duke University Health System, especially the Myeloma Faculty, Drs. Long, Kang, Choi and Costa. A special thanks to Dr. David Rizzieri and Dr. Nelson Chao for supporting and believing in the success of the multiple myeloma program at Duke. We are particularly grateful to the incredible nurses of the inpatient and outpatient services at Duke – without their dedication we could not provide the quality of patient care that has come to represent the hallmark of our program.

Artist Acknowledgment:

We acknowledge Dorothy J. Swartz for providing artistic support in rendering the cover artwork.

Cristina Gasparetto, MD
Dharshan Sivaraj

© Herzlinde Vancura/Dreamstime.com

CHAPTER 1

Who Gets Multiple Myeloma?

Multiple myeloma (MM), with an incidence of 6.3 per 100,000 Americans per year, is the second most common cancer of the blood after non-Hodgkin's lymphoma. The American Cancer Society estimates that 17,500 men and 12,800 women were diagnosed with multiple myeloma in the United States in 2016. It is estimated that approximately 30,300 new cases of myeloma will be diagnosed in the US in 2017. The chance of developing myeloma increases as people get older, though it occurs infrequently in people under the age of 40 (**TABLE 1-1**).

Multiple myeloma has occasionally been reported in children and is seen only rarely in teenagers. The median age of affected patients is 65 years, and over 20% of patients are older than age 70 when they are diagnosed. In a significant number of cases, multiple myeloma is preceded by a premalignant[1] condition called monoclonal gammopathy of undetermined significance (MGUS).[2] The incidence of developing MGUS increases with age, approaching 10% in people over the age of 80. The increased incidence observed with age is likely due to a multistep transformation process resulting

---

1 Premalignant refers to a precancerous condition.
2 Monoclonal gammopathy of undetermined significance (MGUS) is a generally asymptomatic plasma cell disorder characterized by low levels of monoclonal protein present in the blood and/or urine (see Chapter 3).

TABLE 1-1 Incidence of Multiple Myeloma Cases by Age*

Age at Time of Diagnosis	Incidence – All Races
Under age 20	0.0
Between 20 and 34	0.6
Between 35 and 44	2.9
Between 45 and 54	10.8
Between 55 and 64	23.3
Between 65 and 74	29.2
Between 75 and 84	24.1
Above age 85	9.2

*Rates are per 100,000 and are age adjusted to the 2000 US Standard Population.
Data from National Cancer Institute. Cancer stat facts: Myeloma. Surveillance, Epidemiology, and End Results Program. https://seer.cancer.gov/statfacts/html/mulmy.html. n.d. Accessed September 22, 2017.

from multiple oncogenic mutations.[3] Over the last 15 to 20 years, however, the number of people diagnosed who are younger than 55 years old has increased, for reasons that remain unclear. Multiple myeloma presents in all races and all geographic locations but is slightly more frequent in men than in women and twice as frequent in blacks than in whites (**TABLE 1-2**).

The incidence is similar in American Indians/Alaska natives, Hispanics, and whites, but is lower in Asians. In black men, myeloma is one of the leading causes of cancer deaths. As of current knowledge, we do not understand what causes this distribution, nor do we know what causes the condition. However, racial differences in the incidence of myeloma and the occurrence of familial[4] myeloma

3 Oncogenic mutations are changes in a normal gene that, under certain situations, can transform a cell into a tumor cell.
4 Familial refers to occurring within a family.

TABLE 1-2 Incidence of Multiple Myeloma per 100,000 in US Population, by Race/Ethnicity and Sex*

Race/Ethnicity	Men	Women
All races	8.3	5.2
White	7.8	4.6
Black	15.9	11.4
Asian/Pacific Islander	4.7	3.2
American Indian/ Alaska native	5.0	5.2
Hispanic	7.7	4.9

*Rates are based on cases diagnosed in 2010–2014 from 18 geographic areas.
Data from National Cancer Institute. Cancer stat facts: Myeloma. Surveillance, Epidemiology, and End Results Program. https://seer.cancer.gov/statfacts/html/mulmy.html. n.d. Accessed September 22, 2017.

suggest that genetic factors are involved. For example, the incidence of myeloma in Chinese and Japanese individuals who have moved to the US is as low as it is in their native countries, suggesting that the incidence is determined largely by genetic factors rather than environmental factors.

The search for the cause of myeloma is ongoing and several possible sources are currently being debated. The first is that something in the environment causes it. The first cases of myeloma reported in the medical literature were described at the beginning of the Industrial Revolution, when synthetic dyes and other organic chemicals were first introduced into the environment. A number of studies have suggested that exposure to pesticides, hair dyes, heavy metal, rubber manufacturing materials, benzene, wood, leather, or petrochemicals increases the risk of developing myeloma, but none have been conclusively demonstrated as a cause.

Several clusters of myeloma occurring in the same geographic location suggest that the environment may be involved. From 1989 through 1992, for example, an excess of myeloma cases was reported in the town of Decatur, Illinois. A study found no occupational cause, but did find an association between an increased risk of developing myeloma and having lived on a farm for some time. Exposure to Agent Orange during the Vietnam War has also been suggested as increasing the risk of myeloma, but there too, the evidence is not conclusive. Several studies of Japanese atomic bomb survivors, radiologists, radium dial workers, and nuclear power plant workers have suggested that radiation exposure might be a predisposing factor in the development of myeloma. Living near nuclear power facilities, however, does not appear to be associated with myeloma.

While all of these studies and observations are provocative, none has conclusively confirmed that an environmental factor or living in a certain place, such as a farm with high pesticide exposure, causes multiple myeloma. Skeletal changes characteristic of multiple myeloma have been found in Egyptian mummies dating back to approximately 1500 to 500 BCE, suggesting that myeloma afflicted people prior to the existence of many of the environmental factors summarized above, and that other factors may be involved. One alternative factor that could be implicated in myeloma is a virus. For example, patients with human immunodeficiency virus (HIV) infections have a 4.5-fold increased risk of developing myeloma. HIV probably does not cause myeloma directly but may contribute to the development of the disease through its effects on the immune system. The fact that the overwhelming majority of people with myeloma do not have HIV indicates that this virus is not an important causative agent.

Another virus that was hypothesized to play a more direct role in causing myeloma is the human herpesvirus 8 (HHV-8), also known as Kaposi's sarcoma-associated herpesvirus (KSHV). This virus has been found in the immune cells of a cohort of patients with early stage myeloma, implying that it may be related to the development of the disease. Of interest, the KSHV/HHV-8 virus produces a protein that is homologous to human interleukin-6 (IL-6).

Interleukin-6 is a cytokine[5] produced by the cells of the immune system that promotes the growth of myeloma cells and stimulates the bone reabsorption that is characteristic of the disease. However, the association between KSHV/HHV-8 and myeloma is controversial, and it remains far from clear whether this virus, or any virus, plays a direct role in the development of myeloma.

Another suggested cause of myeloma is prolonged stimulation of the immune system by repeated infections or autoimmune disease. A few studies have reported an association of myeloma with allergies and diabetes, while other studies have not found or have excluded these associations. Additionally, some studies have suggested an increased incidence of myeloma in patients with rheumatoid arthritis. Other lifestyle factors such as diet, cigarette smoking, and alcohol consumption have yet to be fully explored for associations with multiple myeloma.

Rarely—in approximately 3 cases per 1000—myeloma occurs in several members of the same family. For example, multiple myeloma has been reported in clusters of two or more first-degree relatives (siblings, or parents and children), in identical twins, and in four members spanning three generations in one family. In France, the Myeloma Intergroup identified ~20 families where the risk of developing myeloma is as high as 5%. In some families with multiple cases of MM, the age at diagnosis decreases in successive generations, suggesting that a phenomenon termed genetic anticipation may be involved. Genetic anticipation in an inherited disease is characterized by intensified clinical severity and/or earlier age of onset with each succeeding generation. Anticipation has been described in familial acute leukemia and other blood cancers and more recently in familial myeloma, although the mechanism for it remains unclear. Also, individuals with familial MM appear to show increased susceptibility to other blood cancers, as well as to solid tumors. This suggests that some people may be born with a genetic predisposition to developing myeloma, though the nature of the predisposition remains unknown. The vast majority of people

---

5 Cytokines are a broad category of small proteins implicated in cell signaling.

diagnosed with myeloma, however, do not have a family history of the disease, and the chance that a child of someone with myeloma will also develop it is slight. Because only a small proportion of all cases of myeloma are familial, a genetic predisposition alone is probably not significant enough to cause myeloma.

Most likely, a combination of factors contributes to the development of myeloma. For example, some people may have a familial and/or nonfamilial genetic predisposition for myeloma, but not develop the disease unless they are exposed to a critical environmental factor such as a chemical or virus at a particular time. It also remains possible that there are many different types of myeloma, each with different causes and varying behaviors. Thus, there may never be a single answer as to why people develop this disease. Medical science is just developing the tools to sort out these questions and to find answers about who develops myeloma and why. Eventually, these answers will lead to more effective preventative measures, diagnostic tests, and treatments—perhaps even a cure.

CHAPTER 2

What Is Multiple Myeloma?

Multiple myeloma (MM) is a blood cancer character-ized by the uncontrolled growth and accumulation of a clone of mature and immature plasma cells[1] in the bone marrow (termed intramedullary disease) and in some pa-tients, in other organs or tissues (extramedullary). Multiple my-eloma is classified as a plasma cell dyscrasia (PCD), which refers to a broad spectrum of diseases characterized by clonal prolifer-ation[2] of malignant cells producing monoclonal immunoglobu-lins.[3] PCD is an umbrella term for a host of diseases that include monoclonal gammopathy of undetermined significance (MGUS), smoldering or indolent multiple myeloma (SMM),[4] Waldenstrom's

---

1 Plasma cells are a type of specialized cells responsible for the production of immune proteins called antibodies.
2 Clonal proliferation refers to the process of cell division or multiplication of one type of cell.
3 Monoclonal immunoglobulins (antibodies) are homogeneous pro-teins produced by plasma cells that recognize and bind to foreign substances in the body, thus aiding in their elimination. Those produced by malignant plasma cells serve no function other than to damage tissues in the body.
4 Smoldering (indolent) myeloma is a form of myeloma that presents no clinical symptoms of disease. Also termed *asymptomatic myelo-ma*, or *early stage myeloma* (see Chapter 3).

macroglobulinemia (WM),[5] POEMS syndrome,[6] plasmacytoma,[7] heavy-chain disease,[8] light-chain disease,[9] amyloidosis,[10] multiple myeloma, and plasma cell leukemia (PCL).[11]

Normal plasma cells are part of the immune system and produce immunoglobulins that help fight infections and/or other diseases. Malignant plasma cells, because of their large quantities, secrete an excessive amount of immunoglobulin (which we refer to as M-component or paraprotein) that accumulates in the blood and/or in the urine. Moreover, the immunoglobulin does not perform its normal function of combatting infection. The immunoglobulin secreted by malignant plasma cells can be an intact immunoglobulin—IgG, IgA, IgM, IgD, or IgE (refer to Table 3.1)—or only the κ or λ light-chain component[12] (also called the Bence Jones protein). Rarely, in less than 0.1% of cases, malignant plasma cells do not secrete immunoglobulins, and these

---

5 Waldenstrom's macroglobulinemia (WM) is not a form of myeloma. It is a rare type of cancer that affects plasma cells, causing the production of excessive amounts of IgM protein.

6 POEMS syndrome is an extremely rare plasma cell disorder involving several components including the presence of a monoclonal plasma cell disorder and peripheral neuropathy, organ involvement, and skin abnormalities, among others.

7 Plasmacytoma is a malignant plasma cell tumor growing within the skeleton (solitary plasmacytoma of bone) or within soft tissue (extramedullary plasmacytoma).

8 Heavy-chain disease refers to a plasma cell disorder characterized by the deposition of pieces of immunoglobulin heavy chains in organs (most commonly the kidneys, liver, and heart).

9 Light-chain disease is a plasma cell disorder characterized by the uncontrolled overproduction of immunoglobulin light chains by malignant plasma cells that are subsequently deposited in various organs, always including the kidneys (the liver, heart, small intestine, spleen, skin, nervous system, and bone marrow can also be implicated).

10 Amyloidosis is a disease characterized by the deposition of cross-linked light chains in various organs and tissues.

11 Plasma cell leukemia is an aggressive malignancy that is characterized by circulating plasma cells in the peripheral blood.

12 Light-chain component refers to a particular subunit of an immunoglobulin. The two variations of light-chain component are κ and λ.

are termed nonsecretory myelomas. In patients with myeloma, the excessive amount of immunoglobulin may cause the blood to become viscous (hyperviscosity syndrome). The light-chain portion of the intact immunoglobulin can be filtered through the kidneys and/or can deposit in the kidneys and damage them, causing renal insufficiency. Additionally, the indiscriminate growth of the malignant plasma cells in the bone marrow causes a unique form of bone destruction, which commonly leads to bone pain and the classic osteolytic bone lesions[13] observed in X-rays. The bone damage causes the bone to weaken, and some patients with myeloma will experience spontaneous bone fractures or fracture following only a minor injury. Other common clinical manifestations of multiple myeloma are anemia,[14] elevated calcium (hypercalcemia), and recurrent infections due to the impaired production of normal immunoglobulins.

▶ History of Multiple Myeloma

Multiple myeloma is an ancient disease. Much of the history of this disease was documented by Dr. Robert A. Kyle of the Mayo Clinic. The text below is drawn heavily from his published work (R.A. Kyle. History of multiple myeloma, *Blood* 2008*). As previously mentioned, skeletal symptoms of the disease have been described in Egyptian mummies. Dr. William Macintyre, a consultant and physician in the Metropolitan Convalescent Institution and the Western General Dispensary in St. Marylebone, London, reported the first case of myeloma in the medical literature in 1850. Dr. Macintyre described one of his patients as follows:

> *"Mr. M., a highly respectable tradesman, age 45, placed himself under my care on the 30th of October, 1845. He was then confined to the house by excruciating pains of the chest, back, and loins, from which he had been suffering, more or less, for upwards to twelve months).*

---

13 Osteolytic bone lesion refers to an area of bone loss in the skeleton that can be identified as a "hole" on an X-ray.
14 Anemia is a deficiency of red blood cells or of hemoglobin in the blood.

Because the patient was suffering from edema[15] of the lower legs, Dr. Macintyre examined the urine and found it to "abound in animal matter." He then sent a urine sample to Dr. Henry Bence Jones, an accomplished chemical pathologist in London with the following message:

> *"Dear Doctor Jones, the tube contains urine of very high specific gravity. When boiled it becomes slightly opaque. On addition of nitric acid, it effervesces, assumes a reddish hue, and becomes quite clear; but as it cools, assumes the consistence and appearance which you see. Heat reliquifies it. What is it?"*

Dr. Bence Jones concluded that the "animal matter" was a protein and he was the first to associate this phenomenon in other cases of myeloma. Because of that, the term *Bence Jones proteinuria* (BJP) is still used to identify the protein in the urine in patients with myeloma and other plasma cells dyscrasias. Dr. J. von Rustizky introduced the term *multiple myeloma* in 1873 in a report of an autopsy of a 47-year-old man who had presented with a tumor in the right temple. Upon further investigation, Dr. von Rustizky noted eight additional separate tumors of the bone marrow and termed them *multiple myeloma* (in Russia, *Rustizky's disease* is still often used). Wilhelm Waldeyer first coined the term *plasma cell* in 1875 and 20 years later Tamás Marschalkó described plasma cells as large oval cells with an eccentric nucleus,[16] large dark cytoplasm,[17] and a pale perinuclear area[18] termed the *hof*. In 1900, James Wright tied these various observations together by suggesting that multiple myeloma originated from these plasma cells. The discovery of X-rays helped to facilitate the diagnosis of myeloma, as bone involvement characteristic of the disease could be identified. In 1928, Charles

---

15 Edema refers to swelling caused by excess fluid trapped in body tissues. *Kyle RA, Rajkumar SV. Multiple myeloma. *Blood.* 2008;111(6):2962–2972 and Kyle RA, Steensma DP. History of multiple myeloma. *Recent Results Cancer Res.* 2011;183:3–23.
16 Nucleus refers to a membrane-bound structure containing the cell's genetic material.
17 Cytoplasm is the fluid that fills a cell, containing many of the cell's structures.
18 Perinuclear area refers to the area just around the nucleus of a cell.

Geschickter and Murray Copeland, after reviewing more than 400 case of multiple myeloma reported in the literature since 1848, described the six major symptoms of the disease: *back pain, pathologic fractures, multiple bone involvement, anemia, Bence Jones proteinuria,* and *renal insufficiency.* In 1928, W. A. Perlzweig first reported that an unusual protein could also be detected in the blood of a patient with multiple myeloma. Lewis Longsworth introduced the use of electrophoresis[19] to identify the MM protein, in 1939. Leonhard Korngold and Rose Lipari in 1956 demonstrated the exact chemical composition of the proteinuria as the light-chain portion of the immunoglobulin molecule. In 1962, approximately 100 years after the first case of multiple myeloma was reported, Daniel Bergsagel, then at the MD Anderson Cancer Center, treated 24 patients with MM with a new chemotherapeutic agent called melphalan[20] and reported significant improvement in 8 and minor improvement in 6. This strategy marked both a significant milestone and a major advance in the treatment of myeloma.

Since its introduction in 1962, melphalan has been incorporated in the treatment for the majority of patients with myeloma. More recently, the introduction of newer medications such as thalidomide, lenalidomide, and bortezomib (see Chapter 4) in conjunction with high-dose therapy[21] and stem cell rescue[22] have had a tremendous impact on the life of patients with MM, providing new options for those with resistant disease and also for those with newly diagnosed MM. We have learned that with such approaches, bringing myeloma closer to resemble a chronic disease rather than a terminal illness

---

19 Electrophoresis is a laboratory technique used to separate certain molecules, including proteins, based on their size.
20 Melphalan is a chemotherapy drug used in the treatment of cancer, primarily multiple myeloma (see Chapter 4).
21 High-dose therapy refers to the use of high doses of chemotherapy most commonly in preparation for a stem cell transplant (see Chapter 5).
22 Stem cell rescue refers to the use of a stem cell transplant after subsequent administration of high-dose therapy (see Chapter 5).

is possible. Additionally, understanding the biology of malignant plasma cells, unmasking MM drug resistance, and discovering new targets for drug development are keys to a potential cure.

The second portion of this chapter will focus on the biology of the disease, the structure of immunoglobulins, the development of plasma cells and the production of immunoglobulins, the role of the bone marrow microenvironment in the pathogenesis[23] of multiple myeloma, tumor angiogenesis,[24] and myeloma bone disease.

▶ Immunoglobulins (Antibodies)

Immunoglobulins are antibodies[25] that identify and mark foreign material in the body for processing by the immune system. The immunoglobulin (Ig) molecule is shaped like a Y and consists of two identical heavy chains, and two identical light chains (**FIGURE 2-1**). The heavy chain and light chain are composed of a variable region and a constant region. The variable region in the heavy chain is derived from three distinct gene segments—the variable (V), diversity (D), and joining (J) region sequences. The light chain derives from the light-chain segments (variable κ or λ) and the joining segment genes.[26] Immunoglobulin heavy- and light-chain genes also contain three hypervariable or complementarity-determining regions (CDRs).[27] While our bodies generate over 10 billion different immunoglobulins, we possess less than 30,000 genes that encode them. In order to

---

23 Pathogenesis refers to the cellular events, reactions, and mechanisms that contribute to the development of a disease.
24 Angiogenesis is the stimulation of new blood vessel formation to supply a tissue or tumor.
25 Antibody is another name for an immunoglobulin. Antibodies are produced by plasma cells in order to identify and neutralize foreign pathogens.
26 Joining segment genes are genes (regions of DNA) that code for the molecules that function to join the variable and constant regions of immunoglobulins.
27 Complementarity-determining regions (CDRs) are portions of an immunoglobulin that bind to an antigen. They are the most variable portions of the immunoglobulin.

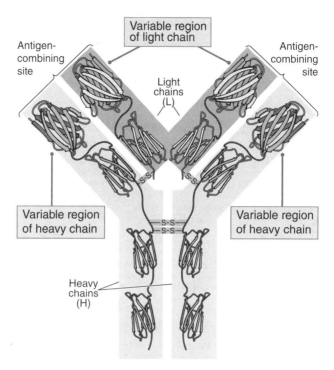

FIGURE 2-1 Immunoglobulin

produce this wide diversity, immunoglobulin-encoding genes are able to rearrange through a mechanism known as VDJ recombination.[28]

Heavy-chain genes undergo rearrangement before the light-chain genes, and the κ precedes the λ rearrangement. B cells, which are types of white blood cells responsible for producing antibodies, can produce five different types of heavy chains (G, A, M, D, and E). Thus, there are five different immunoglobulin classes or types (IgG, IgA, IgM, IgD, and IgE). Plasma cells are a common type of differentiated B cell,[29] and can produce only two types of light chains (κ and λ). In addition, there are four subtypes of IgG (IgG1, IgG2, IgG3, and IgG4) and two subtypes of IgA (IgA1 and IgA2). IgA and IgM immunoglobulins are larger than the other immunoglobulins

---

28 VDJ recombination is a unique process of genetic recombination that results in an extremely diverse population of immunoglobulins produced by our plasma cells.

29 Differentiated B cells refer to either plasma cells or memory cells, which are derived from B cells.

and thus, when present in high quantity in the blood of a patient, they can cause symptoms associated with increased blood thickness. IgM is a pentamer, with five Ys joined together, and IgA is a dimer with two Ys joined together. Symptoms due to thick blood, or *hyperviscosity syndrome* include: fatigue, blurred vision, drowsiness, vertigo, chest pain, and bleeding tendency. Hyperviscosity syndrome occurs more often in immunocytoma (Waldenstrom's macroglobulinemia, an IgM disorder) and less frequently in patients with IgA or IgG multiple myeloma types.

Idiotype

Both the heavy chains and the light chains are composed by sequences of repeating amino acids[30] or blocks (structural domains). Both the heavy and the light portion of the immunoglobulin have a "constant region" and a "variable region" (Figure 2-1). The sequence of amino acids in the constant portion is always the same, while the sequence of the amino acids in the variable portion is always different, with respect to each different immunoglobulin. The heavy and the light chains in the immunoglobulin have the variable regions close together to form a groove or *idiotype*. The idiotype is the region where the antigen[31] binds. During one's life, a person comes in contact with thousands of antigens and each antigen stimulates the production of over a thousand different antibodies. Therefore, in a healthy individual there is an enormous diversity of immunoglobulins, or *polyclonal* immunoglobulins with different idiotypes. That is true in patients with myeloma as well, but in addition there is a large amount of a single immunoglobulin, or fragment of one, called the *monoclonal* antibody referred to as the M protein. The M protein can be detected in the blood and/or urine of patients with myeloma using a technique called electrophoresis (please refer to Chapter 3). The M protein produced by the malignant cells has the same heavy-chain type, the same light-chain type, and the same idiotype. The idiotype can

---

30 Amino acids are the molecular building blocks of proteins.
31 Antigen is any substance that stimulates the body to produce antibodies against it. Can either be a foreign substance or a substance formed within the body such as a bacterial toxin or a malignant tissue cell.

serve as a tumor marker to follow response to therapy and disease progression. The idiotype can also potentially be used as a target to build and create specific tumor vaccines to fight myeloma.

▶ Plasma Cells

Mature plasma cells are large (20 micrometers in diameter), oval-shaped cells that contain an eccentric bilobed[32] or multilobed[33] nucleus, as well as a cytoplasm that stains blue or dark gray (termed *basophilic*) with commonly used pathology reagents.[34] Plasma cells are found in the lymph nodes and bone marrow, but those residing in the bone marrow are the main source of the serum immunoglobulins. Plasma cells comprise from 0.2%–2.8% of the bone marrow white blood cells,[35] and they are rarely found in the peripheral blood.[36] All lymphocytes,[37] including plasma cells, derive from a common lymphoid progenitor,[38] which has the capacity to develop into T,[39] B, or natural killer (NK)[40] cells. The earliest committed B cell is called the *B-cell progenitor cell* or *null cell*. The B-cell progenitor cell needs to undergo several stages of differentiation[41] prior to becoming a mature plasma cell, which can produce specific

---

32 Bilobed refers to consisting of two lobes, or "roundish" divisions.
33 Multilobed refers to consisting of an excess of two lobes.
34 Pathology reagents are chemicals used in laboratory examinations of body tissues.
35 White blood cells are the cells of the immune system that are involved in protecting the body against malignant foreign substances as well as infectious disease.
36 Peripheral blood refers to circulating blood in the body.
37 Lymphocytes are a class of white blood cells in our immune system that help fight infection and protect the body against diseases.
38 Lymphoid progenitor cells can be thought of as parent cells that create new lymphocytes.
39 T cells are a type of lymphocyte that plays a major role in the immune system by acting to identify and destroy infectious agents.
40 Natural killer (NK) cells are a type of lymphocyte that plays a major role in the host-rejection of both virally infected cells and tumors.
41 Differentiation is the process by which unspecialized cells take on certain characteristics and reach their specialized form and function.

antibodies. Subsequent stages include the *pro-B cell,* the *pre-B cell,* the *immature B cell,* the *virgin or mature B cell,* the *activated B cell,* the *B lymphoblast,* the *plasma cell,* or the *memory cell.* In humans new B cells are generated throughout life. During gestation,[42] the steps of plasma cell maturation take place in the liver and thereafter occur in the bone marrow. During the early steps of maturation, or *antigen-independent development,* B cells do not require any interaction with foreign antigens. Subsequently, during the *antigen-dependent phase,* B cells must interact with foreign antigens and/ or regulatory T cells[43] in order to differentiate into either plasma cells or memory cells.[44]

Antigen-Independent Phase

Early committed B-cell progenitors express a type of surface receptor protein[45] known as CD19 and undergo rearrangement of immunoglobulin heavy chain. Early B cells will then express a complex of an immunoglobulin heavy chain together with a surrogate light chain.[46] This step is followed by a similar rearrangement of a κ or λ light-chain gene. The first immunoglobulin produced and expressed on the surface of an immature B cell is IgM. Immature B cells then leave the bone marrow, circulate in the blood, and complete their development in the spleen. At this stage of maturation, B cells are called mature resting or virgin B cells and they acquire the ability of expressing surface IgD in addition to IgM.

---

42 Gestation refers to the time period between conception and birth of a newborn.

43 Regulatory T cells are a subgroup of T cells that function to modulate the immune system and prevent autoimmune disease.

44 Memory cells are a class of white blood cells whose function results in a more efficient and rapid response to a previously encountered pathogen.

45 Surface receptor proteins are special proteins that communicate signals between the cell and its outside environment.

46 Surrogate light chain is a protein similar to an immunoglobulin light chain that associates with immunoglobulin heavy chains to form early B-cell receptors.

Antigen-Dependent Phase

When virgin or mature B cells interact with foreign antigens and/or regulatory T cells, they become activated and proliferate to give rise to either *plasma cells* or *memory cells*. It is unclear why some mature B cells will become plasma cells and others memory cells. Memory cells have a long life span (years to decades in some cases) and they are responsible for the secondary immune response.[47] Memory cells can proliferate and generate a plasma cell more rapidly than a mature B cell can.

The immature or pre-switched B cells express surface IgM and IgD, while the post-switched or mature B cells may express IgA, IgG, IgD, or IgE. Mature B cells travel to the bone marrow where they adhere and interact with stromal cells[48] and subsequently differentiate into plasma cells.

Malignant Plasma Cell Transformation

For myeloma to develop, genetic mutations in a single cell disrupt this orderly developmental process leading to uncontrolled growth and proliferation. However, the stage in plasma cell development where these mutations occur and malignant transformation begins is currently unknown. Some recent evidence suggests that the transformation may in fact occur in early stages of B-cell development, giving rise to the notion that there may be rare primitive *myeloma stem cells* that generate a large number of mature myeloma plasma cells. If myeloma stem cells are ultimately proven to exist, this could have important implications for the diagnosis and treatment of myeloma, as they may have biologic properties that are different from the much more numerous mature myeloma plasma cells. Consequently, to cure myeloma it may be necessary to understand the biology of these rare myeloma stem cells and more importantly, find ways to eliminate them so that they cannot regenerate the disease.

---

47 Secondary immune response refers to the body's immune reaction to a previously encountered antigen. Characterized by being more rapid than the primary immune response.
48 Stromal cells are the connective tissue cells of an organ.

▶ Myeloma Pathogenesis

The development of myeloma is the result of a progression that nearly always begins with a nonmalignant precursor state termed a *monoclonal gammopathy of undetermined significance* (*MGUS*), which is characterized by a low percentage of myeloma cell growth in the bone marrow and the absence of organ involvement or bone destruction (please refer to Chapter 3). When the malignant plasma cell percentage in the bone marrow exceeds 10%, this disease state transitions into either a condition known as smoldering myeloma, or into clinically defined symptomatic myeloma.

The rate of progression to multiple myeloma from MGUS is approximately 1% per year. This progression is potentially influenced by several factors including intraclonal heterogeneity, changes in the bone marrow microenvironment, and the presence of other systemic factors. The intermediate stage between MGUS and symptomatic myeloma is defined as smoldering myeloma (see Chapter 3). The rate of progression from smoldering myeloma to symptomatic myeloma is approximately 10% per year for the first 5 years after diagnosis. A final stage of progression after symptomatic myeloma can be plasma cell leukemia (PCL), which arises as a result of myeloma resistance to therapy as well as clonal evolution.[49] This condition is characterized by the spilling of plasma cells (>20%) from the bone marrow into the bloodstream, which can lead to the creation of plasmacytomas outside the bone marrow around the body. Significant research is being devoted to better understand the pathogenesis of all stages of this disease, including the precursor (MGUS/smoldering MM), symptomatic (MM), and terminal (PCL) stages. Please refer to Chapter 3 for a more detailed description of these disease stages.

The bone marrow (BM) environment plays a major role in the pathogenesis of multiple myeloma. In fact, it is extremely difficult to grow normal as well as malignant plasma cells in

---

49 Clonal evolution theory is the hypothesis that multiple myeloma arises from normal plasma cells that mutate and generate abnormal offspring that themselves also mutate. This results in a branched lineage of genetically varied subpopulations of myeloma cells.

vitro[50] without the support of the BM microenvironment. The BM provides signals to myeloma cells that influence the tumor cell growth, survival, migration, and drug resistance. In multiple myeloma the homeostasis[51] between the cellular, the extracellular, and the liquid compartment[52] is thoroughly disrupted. The association between the bone marrow microenvironment and the pathogenesis of myeloma represents an important field of research. This research could lead to more treatments that interfere with the pathogenesis of MM in the bone marrow microenvironment, slow disease progression, and ultimately help improve patient outcomes and quality of life.

▶ The Bone Marrow Microenvironment

During the adult life, blood cells are continuously produced in the bone marrow. The bone marrow is a soft fatty tissue found inside large bones, such as the chest bone (sternum), the hipbone (pelvis), and the thighbone (femur). The bone marrow microenvironment is composed of hematopoietic stem cells,[53] progenitor cells,[54] immune cells, erythrocytes,[55] bone marrow stromal cells (BMSCs),[56]

---

50 In vitro refers to a process occurring outside a living organism, commonly in a laboratory test tube or culture dish.

51 Homeostasis is the tendency of a system to gravitate towards maintaining internal stability and equilibrium.

52 Liquid compartment refers to the liquid environment of signaling and growth factors within the bone marrow.

53 Hematopoietic stem cells are cells isolated from the blood or bone marrow that give rise to all the other blood cells found in the body.

54 Progenitor cells are descendants of stem cells that can differentiate into other cells but cannot divide indefinitely.

55 Erythrocytes refer to another term for red blood cells, which deliver oxygen to the body's tissues.

56 Bone marrow stromal cells are cells that make up a portion of the bone marrow not directly involved in blood cell production. BSMCs consist of various cell types including fibroblasts, osteoblasts, osteoclasts, and endothelial cells, among others.

osteoclasts (OCLs),[57] osteoblasts (OBLs),[58] and vascular endothelial cells.[59] The bone marrow stromal cells not only directly interact with MM cells, but also secrete growth factors such as interleukin 6 (IL-6), insulin-growth factor-I (IGF-I), vascular endothelial growth factor (VEGF), and tumor necrosis factor-α (TNF-α),[60] which have been implicated in the survival, proliferation, and differentiation of myeloma. MM cells can also secrete inflammatory factors [such as VEGF, basic fibroblast growth factor (BFGF), TNF-α, transforming growth factor-β (TGF-β), and macrophage inflammatory protein 1-α (MIP-1α)] that further augment cytokine production. For example, TNF-α, VEGF, and TGF-β secreted from MM cells enhance IL-6 secretion from the bone marrow stromal cells. IL-6 is an important cytokine in MM pathogenesis. IL-6 induces growth of the MM cells both in vitro and in vivo[61] by stimulation of MM cell division and by prevention of programmed myeloma cell death (apoptosis). Apoptosis is a normal and controlled phenomenon that occurs in a cell's development, involving self-induced death. In myeloma cells, inflammatory cytokine IL-6, among others, has been shown to stimulate the ability of myeloma cells to evade the engagement of apoptosis, leading to uncontrolled growth and resistance to therapy. Novel therapies are therefore designed to target not only the MM cells, but also these microenvironment interactions, as well as to alter the production of cytokines. Ultimately these therapies may help overcome resistance to conventional therapies and improve outcomes for patients.

---

57 Osteoclasts are a type of bone cells that function to break down bone tissue.
58 Osteoblasts are a type of bone cells that build new bone tissue.
59 Vascular endothelial cells are thin, flattened cells that line the inner surfaces of blood vessels.
60 IL-6, IGF-I, VEGF, and TNF-α are growth factors that have been shown to enhance the survival, proliferation, and differentiation of myeloma cells.
61 In-vivo refers to occurring or being performed in a living organism (in contrast to in-vitro).

The BM (bone marrow) vasculature[62] represents a barrier between the BM cells and the peripheral circulation. The BM vasculature is altered in MM and an increase in microvascular density (MVD)[63] correlates with disease progression. The role of tumor angiogenesis or increased blood vessel formation is well established in solid tumors and correlates with tumor growth. A number of studies demonstrate a role for angiogenesis in numerous blood cancers as well, including multiple myeloma.

▶ Tumor Angiogenesis

As myeloma progresses, the number and volume of blood vessels in the bone marrow also increases in a process called *angiogenesis*. As patients with myeloma respond to therapy, the quantity of blood vessels in the bone marrow decreases. Due to this observation, it is now clear that small blood vessels in the bone marrow serve an important role in supporting the growth of myeloma cells. Basic fibroblast growth factor (BFGF) and vascular endothelial growth factor (VEGF) are cytokines produced by the stromal cells and other white blood cells. These substances promote the growth of blood vessels in the bone marrow and play an important role in the growth of myeloma cells as well. Blocking these molecules may also be a key target in attacking multiple myeloma.

One of the major sources of mortality and morbidity for patients with MM results from osteolytic bone lesions or bone destruction throughout the axial skeleton. Osteolytic lesions occur in 70%–80% of patients with MM. These lesions are often associated with debilitating pain and bone fractures. As a consequence of the bone destruction, patients with MM frequently develop elevated levels of calcium in the blood (termed hypercalcemia). Understanding the mechanisms responsible for the bone destruction should lead to novel therapies that can ultimately improve the quality of life for patients with myeloma.

---

62 Bone marrow (BM) vasculature refers to arrangement of blood vessels in the bone marrow.
63 Microvascular density (MVD) refers to the concentration of small blood vessels in a particular area.

▶ Bone Destruction in Multiple Myeloma

The indiscriminate growth of the malignant plasma cells in the bone marrow causes a unique form of bone destruction. Bones in healthy individuals change constantly, breaking down and being rebuilt as part of the living process. Two kinds of cells are important for this process—osteoclasts and osteoblasts. Osteoclasts dissolve or reabsorb the old bone, leaving an empty space. The osteoblasts then fill this empty space with new bone. If the rate of bone renewal does not equal the rate of breakdown, bone loss occurs. In multiple myeloma the bone destruction is caused by an increased number of osteoclasts growing in the vicinity of the myeloma cells. The malignant plasma cells grow within the bone marrow in close contact with stromal cells and produce cytokines that promote the growth and activity of the osteoclasts, while simultaneously impairing the function of the osteoblasts. Some of these cytokines are important to maintain the growth of the malignant plasma cells themselves, and they are also important in the development of tumor drug resistance as mentioned above.

In healthy individuals another substance called RANKL (*r*eceptor *a*ctivator of *n*uclear factor κ-B *l*igand)[64] enhances the growth and activity of osteoclasts. RANKL is kept under control by osteoprotegerin (OPG).[65] The balance between RANKL and OPG is important to bone maintenance. Evidence suggests that in patients with myeloma there is an imbalance between these two substances, RANKL and OPG, and this imbalance also contributes greatly to the bone loss observed in myeloma.

Another potent inducer of osteoclast formation is macrophage inflammatory protein 1-α (MIP-1α).[66] Levels of MIP-1α are elevated in patients with MM and correlates with the presence of osteolytic lesions. The lower activity of osteoblasts observed in patients with

---

64 RANKL is a protein implicated in the regeneration and remodeling of bones.
65 Osteoprotegerin (OPG) is a cytokine with the ability to inhibit the production of osteoclasts.
66 Macrophage inflammatory protein 1-α (MIP-1a) is a molecule implicated in the release of inflammatory cytokines.

MM may also contribute to the development of osteolytic lesions. MM cells directly inhibit the differentiation of osteoblastic cells from mesenchymal cells[67] through cell-to-cell contact and through the secretion of soluble factors such as IL-3 and IL-7, which serve to decrease expression of osteoblast markers as well as inhibit bone formation through the reduction of various promoters[68] involved in osteoblast function. A deeper understanding of the development of MM bone disease will aid the discovery of novel agents that help to restore normal bone remodeling.

▶ Drug Resistance

Drug resistance represents an important aspect of myeloma relapse and disease progression. The presence of drug-resistant subpopulations of cells that are either initially present or arise during the course of treatment is a hallmark of this disease. Taking an evolutionary approach to understanding myeloma can help provide deeper insights into how the disease persists and ultimately relapses, even in the presence of effective therapies. Multiple myeloma cells are heterogeneous (termed intraclonal heterogeneity (ICH)[69]) and thus differ in their biological characteristics and sensitivities to treatments. There is growing evidence that MM patients have many subpopulations of myeloma cells, which can be thought of as continually evolving tumor subclones with variation in their characteristics. While a particular drug may eliminate a large population of MM cells, other subpopulations of cells persist that are either intrinsically resistant or acquire resistance to the therapy via genetic mutations.[70] As these resistant cells divide and repopulate

---

67 Mesenchymal cells is a type of stem cell that differentiate into several other cell types including muscle, bone, cartilage, and fat cells.

68 Promoters are regions of DNA that initiate transcription of a particular gene, which ultimately leads to protein production.

69 Intraclonal heterogeneity (ICH) refers to the presence of variability within cancer cells and cancer cell subpopulations.

70 Mutations are permanent alterations of the DNA (deoxyribonucleic acid) that occur via environmental stimuli, and/or an error during normal cell division.

the bone marrow space, they pass their genetic characteristics onto their progeny,[71] eventually producing a dominant population of drug-resistant cells. We can consider the imposition of a particular drug or treatment as a selective pressure[72] that ultimately favors a more treatment-resistant population of myeloma cells. This is the reason most myeloma patients eventually stop responding to therapy. Due to the omnipresent phenomenon of treatment resistance, multiple drugs with different mechanisms of action are often administrated at the initiation of treatment. The rationale behind this approach is that by giving drugs with different mechanisms of action in combination, there is a reduced likelihood of developing resistance to any single drug used in the combination. Additionally, the use of combination therapies ensures the eradication of as many subpopulations of MM cells as possible.

Unfortunately, myeloma cells have the potential to become cross-resistant to multiple drugs, a situation termed *multiple drug resistance* (MDR). There are several causative processes implicated in both intrinsic and acquired MM drug resistance including the nature of the bone marrow microenvironment, genomic instability,[73] myeloma cancer stem cells,[74] oncogenic mutations, and imbalanced signaling pathways. While the emergence of new MM drugs has significantly improved therapy, the disease eventually develops treatment resistance in nearly all patients. Efforts being made to understand the pathophysiology of MM and the mechanisms by which the disease resists treatment are helping to inform the development of new highly targeted therapies that could prove useful in terms of managing and potentially overcoming MM drug resistance.

---

71 Progeny refers to offspring or descendant that, in this context, is the result of cell division.

72 Selective pressure refers to the extent to which something possessing a certain characteristic is either favored or eliminated due to an environmental restriction.

73 Genomic instability refers to a high frequency of mutations within the chromosomes.

74 Myeloma cancer stem cells are small subpopulations of drug-resistant cancer progenitor cells that are thought to be potentially responsible for disease propagation.

© Herzlinde Vancura/Dreamstime.com

CHAPTER 3

Diagnosis and Staging of Multiple Myeloma

An accurate diagnosis of myeloma is the result of a detailed patient history, physical examination, and diagnostic tests including laboratory analysis and X-rays. This chapter focuses on the diagnostic criteria and classification of multiple myeloma (MM), clinical symptoms, investigational studies, staging systems, and the most relevant prognostic factors for predicting disease outcome and response to therapy.

▶ Diagnostic Criteria and Classification of Multiple Myeloma

Over the years, several systems have been proposed for the classification and the diagnosis of MM. These systems have sought to help distinguish between MGUS, smoldering myeloma, and various stages of early and advanced myeloma in order to help guide decisions about when to start treatment, as well as to provide common definitions for investigators to use when conducting clinical trials. The most commonly used classification systems in the past were the Chronic Leukemia-Myeloma Task Force criteria of Kyle and Greipp, The Southwest Oncology Group (SWOG) of Durie and Salmon, and the British Columbia Cancer Agency (BCCA).

A major criterion in all these systems is the presence of a monoclonal immunoglobulin in the patient's serum[1] and/or urine. Approximately 90% of patients with myeloma secrete a monoclonal immunoglobulin (also termed the M-component[2] or paraprotein[3]) in the serum, and 70%–80% have detectable immunoglobulin fragments, termed Bence Jones protein,[4] in the urine. The M-component is unique for each individual and does not appear to have a specific function. It can be used as a specific *tumor marker*[5] for the diagnosis and follow-up of patients with MM. The most common immunoglobulin type in myeloma is IgG, which is found in approximately 50%–60% of patients (**TABLE 3-1**). IgA is found in 20% of patients, and about 15%–20% of patients with myeloma produce incomplete immunoglobulin κ or λ light chains. IgD and IgE myelomas are very rare. Patients with IgD myeloma usually present with a small monoclonal spike[6] detected in the serum. Bence Jones proteinuria, extramedullary disease,[7] and amyloidosis are frequent in IgD myeloma. Only a few patients with IgE MM have been reported and they present clinical features similar to other MM types. IgM myeloma can occur in rare cases and is distinguishable from Waldenstrom's macroglobulinemia by the absence of enlarged organs (spleen, liver, lymph nodes) and the

---

1 Serum is a clear liquid differing from plasma that can be separated from clotted blood.
2 M-component (or M-spike) refers to an abnormal immunoglobulin that presents in high numbers in patients with certain plasma cell disorders such as myeloma.
3 Paraprotein is another term used in place of the M-component to describe a protein in the serum appearing in large quantities due to a pathological condition.
4 A Bence Jones protein is a monoclonal immunoglobulin light chain found in the urine that is characteristic of multiple myeloma.
5 Tumor marker is a substance in the body fluids or blood that is indicative of an underlying malignancy.
6 Monoclonal spike, also termed M-spike, refers to the large amounts of antibodies or portions of antibodies found in the blood and/or urine of patients with multiple myeloma.
7 Extramedullary disease is also known as extramedullary plasmacytoma; it is a tumor that consists of monoclonal plasma cells that lie outside the bone marrow and separate from the bone.

TABLE 3-1 Types of Monoclonal Immunoglobulins in Patients with Multiple Myeloma

M-Component	% of Patients
IgG	50%–60%
IgA	20%
IgD	0%–1%
IgE	0%–2%
IgM	<1%
Light chain only	20%–30%
Nonsecretory	<1%

Data from Kyle RA et al. Review of 1027 patients with newly diagnosed multiple myeloma. *Mayo Clin Proc*. 2003;78:21-33.

presence of bone destructive lesions. As stated previously, less than 1% of patients do not secrete any M-component in the serum and/or urine; this type of MM is called *nonsecretory myeloma*.

Other disorders associated with monoclonal immunoglobulin production include other B-cell malignancies such as lymphoma[8] and chronic lymphocytic leukemia,[9] Al amyloidosis,[10] crioglobulinemia,[11]

---

8 Lymphoma is a cancer of the lymphatic system, which is part of the body's immune system.
9 Lymphocytic leukemia is a form of cancer of the blood and bone marrow characterized by an abnormal increase in the number of white blood cells.
10 Al Amyloidosis is a disorder characterized by an underlying plasma cell dyscrasia and involves the deposition of amyloid light chains in various organs of the body including the kidneys, heart, liver, gastrointestinal (GI) tract, and nerves.
11 Crioglobulinemia is a condition that causes damage to blood vessels throughout the body.

primary cold agglutinin disease,[12] peripheral neuropathy,[13] dermatological disorders, and infections. Therefore, the presence of an M-component alone is not sufficient to diagnose myeloma, and physicians must conduct additional tests to determine whether the abnormality is due to myeloma or another process. Another commonly used major criteria for the diagnosis of multiple myeloma is the presence of malignant plasma cells greater than or equal to 10% of all the cells in the bone marrow. However, typically plasma cells are not distributed equally throughout the marrow, and therefore the percentage of plasma cells may vary depending on the site of the bone marrow aspirate. The presence of lytic lesions in the bone is a third major criterion for the diagnosis of multiple myeloma. Lytic lesions are holes of varying size in the bones due to bone destruction by the myeloma.

Despite these similarities in the three classification systems described above, each system also had significant discrepancies and concurred completely in the diagnosis of only 64% of patients with MM (Comprehensive Cancer Center, Leiden, Netherland analysis of 157 patients with plasma cell dyscrasias). In 2003, the International Myeloma Working Group (IMWG) published a uniform diagnostic criteria system for the classification and diagnosis of multiple myeloma and other gammopathies[14] (**TABLE 3-2**).

One of the major problems with this classification system is that the diagnosis of myeloma and subsequent initiation of treatment can only be made once overt clinical indications of end-organ damage such as renal insufficiency, anemia, or bone lesions has occurred. By this classification system, patients, even those at a high risk of progressing from the "smoldering" phase, would not be recommended to receive early therapy to prevent organ damage. These criteria were suitable in an era in which treatments caused significant toxicities and the initiation of early treatment showed no real clinical benefit. However,

---

12 Primary cold agglutinin disease is an autoimmune disease that results in the presence of increased quantities of circulating antibodies that target red blood cells.
13 Peripheral neuropathy refers to numbness, pain, and/or tingling; usually in the hands and feet.
14 Gammopathies are disorders of the immune system characterized by abnormally elevated quantities of immunoglobulins in the serum.

TABLE 3-2 IMWG Classification System (2003)	
Plasma Cell Disorder	**Definition**
Multiple myeloma (MM)	1. Presence of M-component in the serum 2. >10% clonal plasma cells in the bone marrow 3. Evidence of organ or tissue damage related to MM: • Serum calcium level >10 mg/L • Renal insufficiency, creatinine >2 mg/dL • Anemia with hemoglobin <10 g/dL • Bone lesions including lytic lesions or osteoporosis with compressive fractures • Amyloidosis • Hyperviscosity syndrome • Recurrent bacterial infections (> two episodes in 12 months)
Monoclonal gammopathy of undetermined significance (MGUS)	1. M-component in serum (<30 g/L) and/or present in urine 2. <10% plasma cells in the bone marrow 3. No evidence of end organ or tissue damage
Asymptomatic (smoldering) multiple myeloma (SMM)	1. M-component in serum (>30 g/L) and/or urine 2. >10% plasma cells in the bone marrow 3. No evidence of end organ or tissue damage
Solitary plasmacytoma	Myeloma can present as an isolated mass in the bone usually in the vertebral column (intramedullary disease) or outside the bone (extramedullary disease) as soft mass most frequently in the upper respiratory tract, parathyroid glands, orbit,[15] lung, spleen, gastrointestinal tract, testes, and skin (extramedullary disease). Two-thirds of patients

(continues)

15 Orbit refers to the cavity in the skull that contains the eyeball.

TABLE 3-2 IMWG Classification System (2003) (*Continued*)	
Plasma Cell Disorder	**Definition**
	with an isolated bone plasmacytoma will eventually develop multiple myeloma at 10 years of follow-up. Patients with an isolated plasmacytoma have: 1. Absent or small M-component 2. Normal bone marrow 3. A biopsy of the mass showing plasma cells 4. No evidence of end organ or tissue damage
Nonsecretory multiple myeloma	1. M-component absent 2. >10% plasma cells in the bone marrow 3. Evidence of end organ or tissue damage

Data from International Myeloma Working Group. Criteria for the classification of monoclonal gammopathies, multiple myeloma and related disorders: A report of the International Myeloma Working Group. *Br J Haematol.* 2003;5:749-757.

with the introduction of newer targeted therapies (see Chapter 4) with much more tolerable side effects, the widespread use of more sensitive imaging techniques, and data suggesting that high-risk patients benefit from early treatment, the criteria published in 2003 were determined to be insufficient. Thus, this classification system was more recently updated to allow for the initiation of treatment in patients who do not meet the prior classification of myeloma, but should be initiated on treatment due to their very high risk of progression to symptomatic disease. With the most recently updated criteria, certain subsets of patients previously defined as smoldering should be treated before organ damage occurs (**TABLE 3-3**).

▶ Clinical Symptoms and Signs of Multiple Myeloma

At time of diagnosis roughly 50%–60% of patients with myeloma have bone pain and 10%–20% have hypercalcemia (elevated calcium in the serum) due to bone destruction. 60%-70% of patients complain

Plasma Cell Disorder	Definition
TABLE 3-3 Revised IMWG Diagnostic Criteria for Multiple Myeloma (2014)	
Multiple myeloma	>10% clonal plasma cells in the bone marrow or biopsy-proven bony or extramedullary plasmacytoma, and any one or more of the following myeloma-defining events (MDE). ■ Evidence of organ or tissue damage related to MM: • Serum calcium level >11 mg/L • Renal insufficiency, creatinine >2 mg/dL • Anemia with hemoglobin <10 g/dL • Bone lesions including lytic lesions or osteoporosis with compressive fractures ■ Biomarkers of malignancy: • ≥60% clonal plasma cells in the bone marrow • Involved/uninvolved serum-free light-chain ratio ≥100 • More than one focal lytic lesion detected by MRI that is ≥ 5 mm
Smoldering myeloma	■ M-component (IgG or IgA) ≥30 g/L or urinary monoclonal protein ≥500 mg per 24/hrs ■ and/or ■ Clonal plasma cells in the bone marrow 10%–60% ■ Absence of any myeloma-defining events listed above, or amyloidosis

MRI = magnetic resonance imaging.

of weakness and fatigue due to underlying anemia, 10%–20% have experienced recurrent infections, and 20%–30% have experienced some weight loss. Less than one-third of patients present with decreased renal function (**TABLE 3-4**).

Bone pain is a common early symptom, particularly in the lower back or ribs. The pain is due to the bone destruction caused by the accumulation of malignant plasma cells in the bone marrow.

TABLE 3-4 Presenting Features of Multiple Myeloma

Symptoms and Signs	Incidence
M-protein serum/urine	97%
Anemia	73%
Lytic bone lesions	66%
Bone pain	53%
Renal insufficiency	19%
Hypercalcemia	13%
Minor or no abnormalities	11%
Hepatomegaly	4%
Amyloidosis	4%
Nonsecretory	3%

Data from Kyle RA et al. Review of 1027 patients with newly diagnosed multiple myeloma. *Mayo Clin Proc.* 2003;78:21-33.

Infiltration of myeloma cells in the spine can weaken the vertebral bones causing them to collapse and impinge on nerves resulting in severe pain, weakness, and numbness.

Bone destruction leads to an increased level of calcium in the blood (hypercalcemia). Increased calcium in the blood can cause a variety of symptoms such as weakness, fatigue, confusion, constipation, increased thirst, increased urine production, nausea, vomiting, and loss of appetite. Elevated calcium can also cause kidney problems. The atypical growth of malignant plasma cells in the bone marrow can cause suppression of the normal red blood cells through an inflammatory process, leading to anemia. Patients with anemia are usually tired and fatigued, may appear pale, and can also experience shortness of breath.

Recurrent bacterial infections as a result of the impaired immune system are also a common presentation of MM. The most common infections are those of the respiratory tract such as bronchitis and pneumonia. Infections of the urinary tract and skin are less common but can be observed occasionally.

Approximately one-third of patients with myeloma presents with or develops kidney insufficiency (renal damage). The main cause of renal damage is deposition of Bence Jones protein in the renal tubules.[16] Other causes include dehydration, hypercalcemia, infections, hyperurecemia,[17] and use of nephrotoxic drugs.[18] In persons with renal insufficiency, decreased erythropoietin[19] production in the kidneys can further contribute to anemia.

Peripheral neuropathy, or numbness, tingling, and abnormal sensation of the hands and feet is present in approximately 5% of patients with myeloma. Other neurologic complications of MM include radicular pain,[20] an early sign of spinal cord or nerve root compression due to fractured vertebral bodies or extramedullary extension of myeloma soft-tissue involvement. Meningeal and cerebral involvement is uncommon in MM and only a few cases have been reported.

Less frequently patients with myeloma can present with chest pain, confusion, dizziness, and shortness of breath due to increased thickness of the blood, or *hyperviscosity syndrome*. As previously mentioned, this occurs when the immunoglobulin concentration in the blood is very high, causing the blood to become unusually thick. Rarely, in patients whose plasma cells produce only the light-chain portion of the immunoglobulin, the light chain can combine with other blood proteins to form amyloid protein.[21] Amyloid protein is a starch-like substance that may deposit in tissues and organs, including the heart, kidney, liver, and nerves disrupting their normal function. This complication of myeloma

---

16 Renal tubules are small tubes in the kidneys that collect, secrete, and conduct urine as well as resorb certain components back into the blood.

17 Hyperurecemia refers to the excess of uric acid in the serum.

18 Nephrotoxic drugs are any type of drug that has a poisonous effect on the kidneys.

19 Erythropoietin is a hormone produced by the kidneys that assists in the rate of production of new red blood cells.

20 Radicular pain is a type of pain due to injury or compression to a spinal nerve root that radiates into the lower extremities.

21 Amyloid protein refers to any number of proteins that can deposit into tissues and cause damage.

is called secondary amyloidosis. Coagulation defects that lead to abnormal bleeding are also rare complications of MM.

Often times, asymptomatic patients at diagnosis are discovered to have multiple myeloma during a routine physical examination and/or routine blood testing. The proportion of patients with no symptoms at time of diagnosis (10%–40%) is increasing, suggesting that the diagnosis is now being made earlier. These patients feel healthy until their myeloma progresses to a more advanced stage. In some patients progression might occur early, while in others, after a long period of observation.

▶ Investigational Studies of Multiple Myeloma

The diagnostic tests for multiple myeloma include serum and urine electrophoresis, serum free light chain (SFLC) assay, imaging studies [radiographic skeletal survey or bone survey, magnetic resonance imaging (MRI), computed tomography (CT) scan, positron emission tomography (PET)], and bone marrow aspiration and biopsy. Other laboratory analyses performed at time of diagnosis and relevant for staging, prognoses, and guiding initiation of therapy, include complete blood cell count, blood smear examination, serum chemistries (including calcium, blood urea nitrogen, creatinine, and lactic dehydrogenase), serum B2-microglobulin level, and quantitative serum immunoglobulin level. These terms will be defined and elaborated upon throughout the course of this chapter.

Serum and Urine Protein Electrophoresis

The M-component can be measured in the serum and/or urine using a laboratory test called *protein electrophoresis*. When placed in gel of agarose[22] containing an electrical field, proteins migrate to different zones or regions, depending on size, shape, and charge. The two major proteins in blood are albumin and globulins. Using serum protein electrophoresis these two groups can be separated into five subgroups or zones (albumin, α_1, α_2, β, and γ regions) (**FIGURE 3-1**):

1. **Albumin** is a protein that carries substances in the bloodstream, helps to keep fluid from leaking into tissues, and

---

22 Agarose is a substance used in gels for electrophoresis.

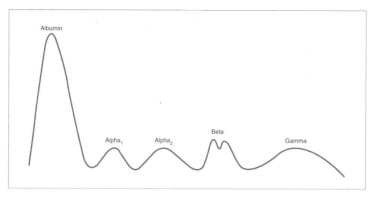

FIGURE 3-1 Normal pattern for serum protein electrophoresis

Reproduced from O'Connell, TX. Understanding and interpreting serum protein electrophoresis. Am Fam Physician. 2005;71(1), 105-112. http://www.aafp.org/afp /2005/0101/p105.html.

contributes to tissue growth and healing. More than half of the total protein in the serum of a normal individual consists of albumin.

2.   **Globulins** can be divided into three fractions based on their electrophoretic mobility.[23] Most of the α and β globulins are synthesized in the liver, whereas γ globulins are produced by lymphocytes and plasma cells in lymphoid tissue.

3. α globulins consist of α_1 and α_2 globulins.

    a. α_1 **globulins** include α_1 antitrypsin,[24] α_1 antichymotrypsin,[25] orosomucoid (acid glycoprotein),[26] serum amyloid A,[27] and α_1 lipoprotein (HDL).[28]

---

23 Electrophoretic mobility is the rate of migration of a particular charged particle in electrophoresis.

24 Antitrypsin is a protein whose deficiency is associated with the development of emphysema.

25 Antichymotripsin is a protein that inhibits the activity of certain enzymes called proteases.

26 Orosomucoid is a protein that is believed to be associated with inflammation.

27 Serum amyloid A is a family of proteins whose concentration increases dramatically in response to tissue inflammation and injury.

28 α_1 lipoprotein (HDL) is a group of proteins in the α_1 family that have high density and low molecular weight.

b. α_2 **globulin** includes serum haptoglobin (a protein that binds hemoglobin and prevents its excretion by the kidneys). Various other α globulins are produced as a result of inflammation, tissue damage, autoimmune disorders, or certain cancers.

c. β **globulins** consist of β_1 and β_2 globulins. β_1 globulins include transferrin (binds iron) and hemopexin.[29] β_2 globulins include complement factors[30] 3 and 4, C-reactive protein,[31] plasminogen,[32] β_2 lipoprotein (LDL),[33] hemopexin, β_2-microglobulin,[34] and some proportion of IgA (especially) and IgM. Fibrinogen[35] also migrates in this region.

d. γ **globulins** consist of the immunoglobulins: IgM, IgA, and IgG.

In the majority of patients with multiple myeloma the M-component migrates in the β or γ zone, although monoclonal immunoglobulin can be found anywhere in the electrophoresis separation between the α_1 zone and the post γ region (Figure 3-1). Thus, migration is specific for each type of M-component. The monoclonal immunoglobulin appears as a sharp and well-defined peak and it can be missed when present at very low concentration. Once the abnormal protein has been detected by electrophoresis, its percentage can be determined with respect to the other globulin fractions by scanning

---

29 Hemopexin is a protein in humans that is an indicator of how much heme is present in the blood.

30 Complement factors are proteins that work to assist the function of antibodies in order to eliminate various antigens.

31 C-reactive protein is a protein that is made by the liver and is released into the bloodstream as a result of tissue injury, infection, or inflammation.

32 Plasminogen is an enzyme present in blood that degrades several blood plasma proteins.

33 β_2-lipoprotein (LCL) is a group of proteins in the β_2 family that have low density and high molecular weight.

34 β_2-microglobulin is a small protein found in the blood whose concentration tends to increase in patients with active myeloma.

35 Fibrinogen is a protein that helps to form blood clots.

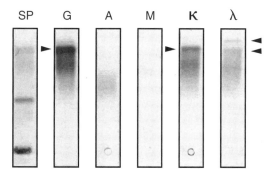

FIGURE 3-2 Example of serum immunofixation

Courtesy of Michael Torbenson, MD and Robert Kelly, PhD.
Retrieved from http://path.upmc.edu/cases/case197.html.

densitometry.[36] Urine electrophoresis functions upon the same principles, and is used to detect and analyze Bence Jones protein as well as assess kidney damage. While Bence Jones protein is not always detected at the time of initial diagnosis, it often appears later. This phenomenon is termed *Bence Jones escape*.

Immunofixation (IFE)

Serum and urine electrophoresis isolate and measure the amount of monoclonal immunoglobulin in a sample but cannot identify the heavy- and light-chain components. Immunofixation (IFE) is used to determine that (**FIGURE 3-2**). After the proteins are separated electrophoretically, specific antisera[37] against each of the heavy and light chains are layered on top of the M-component on the gel. When a specific antiserum reacts with a specific protein, it forms an immune complex[38] that precipitates and becomes fixed into the matrix of the gel. After incubation, the gel is washed to remove all

---

36 Scanning densitometry is a laboratory technique used to measure optical density in light-sensitive materials to determine quantities or percentages of substances.
37 Antisera are blood serum-containing antibodies targeted against specific antigens.
38 Immune complex refers to a molecule formed as a result of the binding of an antigen to an antibody.

the excess antiserum leaving only the antiserum that reacted against a specific protein as a precipitated immune complex.

In Figure 3-2 the first column labeled "SP" refers to the SPEP (serum protein electrophoresis) reading for the patient. The next three columns reflect monoclonal IgG, IgA, and IgM respectively. The last two columns reflect the kappa (κ) and lambda (λ) light chains. When reading a serum immunofixation, the presence of a narrow band with sharp borders indicates the presence of a monoclonal protein. In a normal immunofixation result, there should be an incremental and smooth reduction in color density towards the edges of a broad lane with the absence of a narrow, dense band.

Serum Free Light Chain Assay (Freelite Test)

The heavy and light chains are produced separately within the plasma cell and subsequently join together to form the intact immunoglobulin. In general and for unknown reasons, normal and malignant plasma cells produce more light chains than heavy chains. The extra light chains (free light chains, or FLCs) enter the bloodstream and in normal individuals, a small amount of free light chains is filtered through the kidneys, while a larger amount is reabsorbed back into the bloodstream and is used to form the intact immunoglobulins. The normal levels of κ free light chains are between 3.3 and 19.4 mg/L, while the normal levels of λ free light chains are between 5.71 and 26.3 mg/L. The normal κ/λ ratio is between 0.26 and 1.65. Patients with MM produce an excess amount of one type of light chain, either κ or λ. Therefore, the production of one type of light chain, but not the other, results in an abnormal κ/λ ratio. SPEP and UPEP (urine protein electrophoresis) tests are relatively insensitive to free light chains, but the serum free light chain assay (Freelite assay) can detect even very low levels of free light chains in the serum (**FIGURE 3-3**). The assay is used to diagnose and monitor patients with light-chain multiple myeloma, and patients with amyloid light-chain (AL) amyloidosis. This test is also used to follow patients with MM during the course of their disease, to monitor response to therapy, and to detect earlier relapse. Along with other laboratory tests, it can also be used to monitor patients with MGUS and patients with

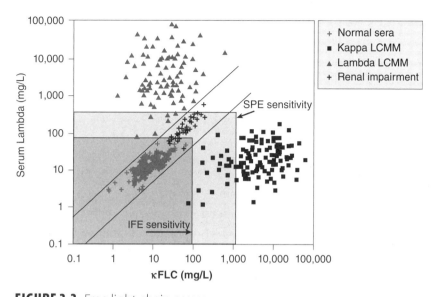

FIGURE 3-3 Free light chain assay

Marian Rollins-Raval, MD, MPH. Retrieved from http://path.upmc.edu/cases/case515/dx.html.

SMM. This test is especially important in diagnosing and tracking patients with light-chain myeloma, a subtype of myeloma in which patients do not present with M-protein in the serum or urine on immunofixation but have a monoclonal free light chain on the SFLC assay. In patients with renal insufficiency due to causes other than MM, both levels of free κ and λ light chains are elevated in the serum as a result of impaired kidney filtration, however the κ/λ ratio remains normal in such patients. In patients with renal failure the FLC ratio can be increased above normal with no other evidence of monoclonal proteins suggesting that in this population the range should be extended (reference range 0.37–3.1).

Heavy/Light Chain Immunoassay (HLC)

Myeloma immunoglobulins (Igs), in particular IgA subtype, may not be accurately measured using the serum protein electrophoresis assay (SPEP). IgA is a larger protein and therefore it migrates slowly in the electrophoresis gel; often it can't be precisely measured due to the interference with normal serum proteins. The heavy/light chain (HLC) immunoassay using specific antibodies can separately distinguish and measure different light-chain types of each immunoglobulin class (IgGκ, IgGλ, IgAκ, and IgAλ), providing accurate quantification of both the involved and uninvolved components of the patient's affected immunoglobulin. The heavy/light chain ratio is becoming a useful tool for screening, monitoring, and risk stratification of patients with multiple myeloma, but also of patients with MGUS and AL amyloidosis.

Complete Blood Cell Count

The complete blood count (CBC) is used to measure the total number of red blood cells, the hemoglobin (substance binds to oxygen in the red cell), the hematocrit (the proportion of red cells in the blood), the total number of white blood cells, the proportion of different white cells, and platelets (substance that clots our blood). Both the myeloma as well as certain medications used to treat it, like chemotherapy, depress the bone marrow and as a result, lower the amount of cells available in the blood. The use of CBC allows for careful monitoring of these counts.

Serum Chemistries

Serum chemistries are used to measure levels of blood urea nitrogen (BUN),[39] creatinine, calcium, albumin, and lactate dehydrogenase (LDH).[40] Increased BUN and creatinine indicate kidney problems. LDH is an indirect measurement of tumor cells burden, and raised concentration is associated with a poor prognosis.

β_2-Microglobulin

β_2-microglobulin is a protein present on the surface of normal and abnormal white blood cells, including plasma cells. The rapid cell turnover characteristic of patients with multiple myeloma and other B-cell malignancies causes the β_2-microglobulin level in the blood to increase. As a result, at time of diagnosis, the level of the β_2-microglobulin

---

39 Blood urea nitrogen (BUN) is nitrogen found in the blood that is produced as a waste product of urea. It serves as a measure of kidney function.

40 Lactate dehydrogenase (LDH) is an enzyme present in nearly all tissues of the body whose concentration in the bloodstream increases in response to cellular damage. Its quantity can be measured to monitor myeloma activity.

often reflects how advanced the disease is and usually correlates with the prognosis. Patients with high level of B_2-microglobulin at time of presentation have a more advanced myeloma. β_2-microglobulin level also rises during exposure to certain viruses, including cytomegalovirus and human immunodeficiency virus (HIV). Because it is normally filtered through the kidneys, patients with kidney insufficiency have high level of β_2-microglobulin in the blood.

C-Reactive Protein

C-reactive protein (CRP) is produced by the liver in response to many inflammatory processes and in response to IL-6. The level of CRP in the blood is therefore elevated in patients with infections, inflammatory diseases, and certain cancers including multiple myeloma. The addition of CRP to MM cells in vitro has been shown to not only stimulate their proliferation and their growth, but also protect MM cells from chemotherapy drugs. In addition, CRP stimulates MM cells to produce more IL-6. A high level of CRP detected in the blood correlates with a more advanced stage myeloma.

Immunoglobulin Profile

This test is used to measure concentration of normal immunoglobulins in the serum (IgA, IgG, IgM, and IgE). In patients with multiple myeloma the production of normal immunoglobulins is generally suppressed, leading to the development of recurrent infections. Serum immunoglobulin concentrations are commonly measured by immunonephelometry[41] or immunoturbidimetry.[42]

Viscosity

Hyperviscosity syndrome is caused by the increased concentration of the M-protein in the blood and also by the molecular characteristic

---

41 Immunonephelometry is a technique used to determine the levels of several blood plasma proteins including the various classes of immunoglobulins.
42 Immunoturbidimetry is another technique used as a tool to determine proteins in the serum that cannot be detected by traditional methods.

(in this case, the tendency to aggregate) of the protein. This complication is more commonly associated with IgM paraproteins but can also occur with IgA or IgG (usually IgG3) paraproteins. Paraprotein (M-protein) concentrations above 30 g/L are often associated with hyperviscosity. The absolute unit of plasma viscosity is in milliPascal seconds (mPa.s). An average plasma viscosity is 1.24 mPa.s at 37°C and can be measured by a variety of techniques.

24-Hour Urine Analysis

A 24-hour urine analysis measures the amount of urine produced in a day, its acidity (pH), and the amount of certain substances in the urine, including proteins. Protein electrophoresis is the only reliable method for the detection of paraproteins in the urine. Once the abnormal protein has been detected, its concentration can be determined by scanning densitometry. IFE (immunofixation) is used to determine the type of the immunoglobulins.

Imaging Studies

A skeletal survey, which is a panel of bone X-rays, is the standard imaging test for patients with multiple myeloma (**FIGURE 3-4**). Osteolytic lesions caused by myeloma cell activity can be viewed as the more translucent circles within the bones on the X-ray.

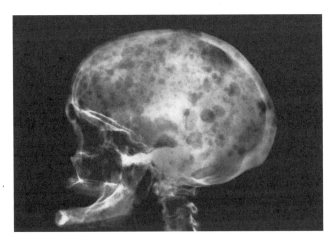

FIGURE 3-4 Skeletal survey of a patient with multiple myeloma

© Photo Researchers/Science Source/Getty Images.

In Figure 3-4, translucent holes can be observed in the humerus and skull bones of a patient. These translucent holes are the osteolytic lesions that form as a result of myeloma cell activity.

Some areas like the ribs, the chest bone, the bones of the shoulders, and the bones of the spine prove difficult to visualize through a skeletal survey and therefore other imaging tests are sometimes required to further evaluate these areas. Additionally, early (underdeveloped) lesions are difficult to visualize through a skeletal survey. The bone needs to lose at least one-third of its mineral structure before the loss can be detected on standard X-ray. One more limitation of the skeletal survey is that when observing an X-ray it is almost impossible to determine if the diffuse bone loss (osteoporosis) is due to myeloma, to aging, or to other causes. Newer imaging studies like computed tomography (CT) and magnetic resonance imaging (MRI) are often used in these circumstances. CT uses a computer to generate three-dimensional X-ray pictures. MRI is a technique that uses magnetic energy to generate images of the bones and surrounding tissues. Hard bone and air appear black and do not give an MRI signal. Soft tissues, spinal fluid, blood, and bone marrow can vary in intensity from black to white based on the MRI settings and quantity of water and fat present in the particular tissue (**FIGURE 3-5**).

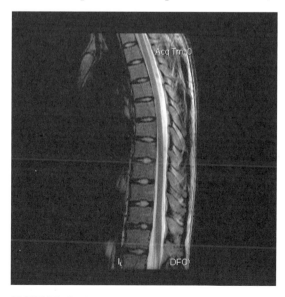

FIGURE 3-5 Thoracic MRI

In Figure 3-5, the thoracic spine (upper-middle back) is depicted through MRI.

MRI is very useful in identifying myeloma involvement of the spine, to determine if new lesions have developed, and to follow response to therapy. MRI is uniquely important to make a diagnosis of spinal cord compression and/or nerve compression or impingement, which can be a result of myeloma cell activity on the bone structure. Patients with extensive disease of the spine detected by MRI have generally a more aggressive myeloma. This imaging technique is also an essential investigation in the diagnosis of solitary plasmacytoma.

Positron emission tomography (PET)[43] scanning using ^{18}F glucose (FDG)[44] is an imaging study to evaluate patients with multiple myeloma. FDG/PET is becoming the preferred diagnostic test to identify occult sites of disease in patients with nonsecretory MM and in patients with a solitary and/or multiple plasmacytomas. PET/CT and whole body MRI are now often used to detect early bone destruction in patients with high-risk smoldering MM and/or early stage MM. It has been demonstrated to be useful in evaluating response to treatment and is thought to have prognostic significance. ^{18}F-FDG PET/CT can help distinguishing between active and inactive disease and therefore is becoming one of the preferred modality to follow patients during the course of their disease. Recently the International Myeloma Working Group (IMWG) coupled this technique with bone marrow minimal residual disease (MRD)[45] to identify patients who had achieved imaging MRD negativity (see below).

Bone Marrow Aspirate and Biopsy

Ultimately the diagnosis of multiple myeloma requires, in part, the identification of greater than or equal to 10% of abnormal plasma

---

43 Positron emission tomography (PET) is a diagnostic test that produces images of the human body, showing differences between healthy and abnormal or cancerous tissues based on the uptake of a radioactive marker.

44 ^{18}F glucose (FDG) is a radioactive marker used in PET scans.

45 Minimal residual disease (MRD) refers to the small quantity of residual tumor that can remain even in patients who have achieved a stringent complete response of their disease.

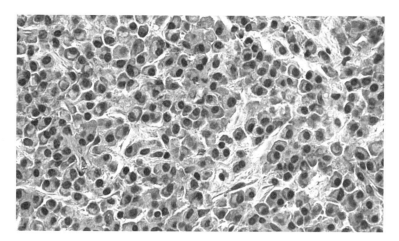

FIGURE 3-6 Malignant plasma cells
© David Litman/Shutterstock.

cells in the bone marrow. The increased number of plasma cells in the marrow can be detected by taking a small liquid sample from the bone marrow (bone marrow aspirate) and a small piece of bone (bone marrow biopsy). Typically bone marrow aspirate and biopsy are taken from the posterior iliac crests (hip bones). Normal plasma cells constitute approximately 1%–5% of the total marrow.

Malignant plasma cells can be distinguished morphologically from normal plasma cells because they are generally associated in sheets or aggregates in the bone marrow, evidencing the uncontrolled growth and producing a mass effect.[46] Malignant plasma cells are often multinucleated (more than one nucleus), and are more immature than normal plasma cells (anaplasia) with prominent nucleoli,[47] reticular chromatin,[48] and high nuclear-cytoplasmic ratios[49] (**FIGURE 3-6**).

---

46 Mass effect refers to the secondary effects of a growing tumor caused by the displacement of surrounding tissue.
47 Nucleolus refers to a small body within the nucleus of a cell that contains protein and genetic material.
48 Chromatin is complexes of DNA and proteins that compose the chromosomes found our cells, arranged in a net-like structure.
49 Nuclear-cytoplasmic ratio refers to the ratio of the size of the nucleus of a cell to the size of the cytoplasm of that cell.

Using immunohistochemical analysis[50] MM cells show light-chain restriction for [κ] and/or [λ], reflecting their clonality. Malignant plasma cells can also be differentiated from normal plasma cells using immunophenotypic markers[51] and flow cytometry analysis.[52] The process of immunophenotyping cells involves the use of CD (cluster of differentiation) markers.[53] CD markers are molecules that are used to help classify white blood cells into subsets. Cells often express many CD markers on their surface with various purposes such as cell adhesion[54] and cell signaling.[55] We use flow cytometry analysis to identify these CD markers. Malignant plasma cells express on their surface CD138. In myeloma, the expressed adhesion molecules are typically $CD38^+$, $CD45^-$, $CD19^-$, and $CD56^+$ while normal plasma cells are $CD19^+$ and $CD56^-$. Overexpression of CD56, the neuronal cell adhesion molecule (N-CAM), is unique to MM cells. We measure serum levels of N-CAM to help distinguish myeloma from other benign monoclonal gammopathies. Furthermore, the interleukin-6 receptor CD126 is expressed only on malignant plasma cells and not on normal plasma cells. Flow cytometry analysis can also be used to detect minimal residual disease (MRD) (see below) in the bone marrow and to detect circulating plasma cells in patients with aggressive myeloma.

Cytogenetic Analysis

Cytogenetics is the science that studies the structure of the chromosomes (structures made up of DNA, of which humans have 23 pairs),

50 Immunohistochemical analysis is a technique used for demonstrating the location and existence of proteins in particular areas of tissue.
51 Immunophenotypic markers are markers used to identify certain cell types existing in a heterogeneous population of cells.
52 Flow cytometry analysis is a technology used to count cells, sort cells, and detect biomarkers with the use of a laser.
53 Cluster of differentiation (CD) markers are cell membrane molecules that are used to stratify white blood cells into classes.
54 Cell adhesion is the process by which cells interact and attach to other cells and substances.
55 Cell signaling refers to a process that is part of an elaborate system of communication that coordinates the actions of cells.

and the lab that performs this test is called the cytogenetics lab. Approximately 30% of patients with myeloma have detectable chromosomal abnormalities using classical cytogenetic testing. One of the major obstacles in performing cytogenetic analysis is that cells need to be dividing and only minorities of the myeloma cells are. To circumvent this problem a test called FISH, which stands for fluorescent in situ hybridization, was developed. With this test, cells can be analyzed even when they are not dividing.

A variety of chromosomal abnormalities can be detected with cytogenetics and FISH. Myeloma cells can have a higher or a lower number of chromosomes than the normal 23 pairs (termed hyperdiploidy and hypodiploidy, respectively). Hypodiploidy is associated with a more aggressive course. Some cells can have numerous other structural chromosome abnormalities. For example, a small portion of the chromosome or the entire chromosome can be missing (this is termed a deletion), or a portion of a chromosome can be found attached to a different chromosome altogether (this is termed a translocation).

One of the most frequent chromosomal abnormality in MM is the deletion of chromosome 13. Lack of chromosome 13, detected by regular cytogenetics, is associated with poor prognosis. This is thought to be due to portions of chromosome 13 encoding for proteins that act as tumor suppressors. Abnormalities on chromosome 1 are also quite common and seem to play an important role in the pathogenesis of multiple myeloma. Many other chromosomes abnormalities have been recently identified using FISH technique, and some appear to be associated with a more aggressive form of myeloma. The most common abnormalities detected by FISH analysis are switch translocations of chromosome 14. To date, the most frequently identified chromosome 14 switch translocations[56] in MM include: t(11;14) in 22%–28%, t(4;14) in 21%, t(8;14) in 4%–10%, t(7;14) in 5%, t(6;14) in 1%, and t(14;16)[57] in 5% of patients. Some of these translocations

56 Switch translocations are chromosomal abnormalities caused by the rearrangement of parts between chromosomes that are not of the same pair.
57 t(_;_) is a notation that refers to the translocation of two chromosomes.

can cause overexpression and activation of proto-oncogenes[58] such as [cyclin D1, fgfr3, c-myc, muml/irf4, and c-maf],[59] and some are associated with poor prognosis.

Microarray Analysis

Microarray analysis is a technology that allows researchers to examine the expression of many thousands of genes. Gene expression refers to the process by which the information in our genetic DNA is converted to a functional product, such as a protein. A gene expression profile (GEP) examines the patterns of many genes in a tissue sample at the same time to examine those that are producing a functional product. By measuring the activity of thousands of genes, a GEP is able to depict a picture of the rate at which those genes are expressed in the tissue sample. Microarray-based GEP analysis estimates the underlying activity of cellular biological pathways that control processes such as apoptosis, cell division, metabolism, and signaling pathways. For example, investigations in myeloma have led to the identification of a number of myeloma subgroups with a defined gene expression profile. GEP is thought to be a means to stratify myeloma patients into risk categories to personalize treatment selection according to the specific biology of their tumors. While further evidence is needed to establish its utility, microarray GEP analysis may have a role in augmenting existing methods of risk stratification or could even serve as a standalone test. Early studies demonstrate that using genetic expression profiling, patients with MM may be classified in a number of groups with different prognoses. This technology has also identified genes that may be important to understand how tumor cells grow, how tumor cells attach to other cells, and how tumor cells develop drug resistance.

---

58 Proto-oncogenes are normal genes, which due to mutations or overexpression, could become an oncogene (a gene that normally guides cell growth whose mutation can result in uncontrolled cell growth, leading to cancer).

59 [cyclin D1, fgfr3, c-myc, muml/irf4, and c-maf] refer to various proto-oncogenes whose mutation and overexpression have been associated with multiple myeloma.

This may also assist in predicting response to treatment, predicting prognosis, and identifying novel targets for future therapy.

Minimal Residual Disease (MRD) Assessment

Minimal residual disease (MRD) refers to the residual cancerous cells that linger in small numbers and evade detection by traditional tests used to measure the quantity of disease burden present after treatment. These residual cancer cells regrow and are responsible for cancer relapse even after a traditionally defined complete remission has been achieved. More recently, technological advances have allowed for identification of the presence or absence of residual myeloma cells (i.e., MRD positivity or MRD negativity) as described below. These tests can be combined with imaging techniques such as FDG/PET to evaluate minimal residual disease both within and outside the bone marrow.

Multi-Parametric Flow Cytometry (MFC)

Multi-parametric flow cytometry (MFC) is a sophisticated test used to count and analyze the size, shape, and properties of individual cells within a heterogeneous population of cells. This technique allows for the measurement of the number and characteristics of myeloma cells taken from a bone marrow sample, and can be used to detect minimal residual disease (MRD). The bone marrow sample is first treated with special fluorescent antibodies and subsequently passed in front of a laser beam. If the antibodies attach to specific antigens on the cells, the cells will emit light. Identifying particular antigens on the surface of the cells allows for identification of the cell type. Some antigens used in MFC to detect malignant plasma cells include CD117, CD28, and CD200, among others. The MFC technique allows for discrimination between myeloma cells and normal plasma cells in bone marrow samples based on variance in antigen expression. Flow cytometry is an extremely sensitive test and can detect MRD to the specificity of 1 myeloma cell in 10,000 to 100,000 total plasma cells within the bone marrow sample. This is particularly useful in monitoring the depth of a patient's remission. One limitation of MFC is the importance of obtaining a bone marrow sample of sufficient quality because a low-quality sample can significantly affect the results. Additionally, the antibody panel[60] used to differentiate myeloma cells from normal plasma cells has yet to be standardized across treatment centers.

Next-Generation Sequencing (NGS)

Next-generation sequencing (NGS) is a technique that is being been explored as an alternative strategy for MRD detection. DNA sequencing refers to the process of determining the precise order of nucleotides[61] within a DNA molecule. NGS refers to a variety of different modern gene sequencing technologies that allow for fast and cheap sequencing of DNA. Next-generation sequencing in the context of multiple myeloma allows for parallel sequencing of the unique clonal immunoglublin heavy chain (IgH) present in each plasma cell and mature B cell. This technique involves performing sequencing at diagnosis to determine the unique IgH rearrangement expressed by the myeloma cell clone. This unique sequence can then later be identified among 100,000 to 1,000,000 amplified IgHs. The sensitivity of NGS-based minimal residual disease (MRD) testing has been reported at 1 in less than or equal to 10^6 cells. Compared to multi-parametric flow cytometry (MFC), NGS is currently more labor intensive, less widely available, and more expensive.

▶ Multiple Myeloma Staging Systems

Staging systems are used to identify how advanced the myeloma is and can help to guide treatment and prognosis. One of the most widely used staging system for multiple myeloma was the Durie-Salmon staging system, first reported in 1975. In this system patients are classified in three major groups (stages I, II, and III) based on the level of the M-component, presence of anemia, hypercalcemia, and the number of bone lesions. Patients are further divided into two additional sub-groups (A and B) based on the level of serum creatinine, which reflects renal function (A: creatinine <2 mg/dL and B: creatinine >2 mg/dL).

---

60 Antibody panel refers to a selection of antibodies selected to detect antigens expressed or not expressed on a particular target cell of interest.
61 Nucleotides are a group of molecules that, when linked together, form the building blocks of our genetic material.

Durie-Salmon Staging System*

Stage 1
- No anemia (hemoglobin $>$10 g/dL)
- A normal level of calcium in the serum ($<$12 mg/dL)
- No evidence of extensive bone destruction (normal X-rays, or a solitary bone lesion)
- Low level of serum M-component (IgG $<$5 g/dL, IgA $<$3 g/dL)

Stage 2
- This stage includes patients who don't fit into stage 1 or stage 3

Stage 3
- Anemia (hemoglobin $<$8.5 g/dL)
- High level of calcium in the serum ($>$12 mg/dL)
- More than three bone destruction lesions
- High level of serum M-component (IgG $>$7 g/dL, IgA $>$5 g/dL, Bence Jones protein $>$12 g/24h)

ISS Staging System

One of the major limitations of the Durie-Salmon staging system was the lack of relevant prognostic indicators. To overcome this problem, the International Staging System (ISS) was proposed in 2003. This system is based on the measurement of serum levels of B_2-microglobulin and albumin. As stated previously, high serum B_2-microglobulin is indicative of high tumor mass and reduced renal function. Low serum albumin in multiple myeloma is a result of inflammatory cytokines like IL-6 secreted by the multiple myeloma microenvironment.**

Stage 1 – Normal albumin $>$3.5 g/dL and low β_2-microglobulin $<$3.5 mg/dL
Stage 2 – Neither stage 1 or/nor stage 3
Stage 3 – β_2-microblublin $>$5.5 mg/dL

---

*Durie BG, Salmon SE. A clinical staging system for multiple myeloma. Correlation of measured myeloma cell mass with presenting clinical features, response to treatment, and survival. *Cancer*. 1975;36(3): 842–854.
**Greipp PR, San Miguel J, Durie BGM, et al. International staging system for multiple myeloma. *J. Clin. Oncol.* 2005;23(15):3412–3420.

R-ISS Staging System

Patients who have ISS stage 3 disease appear to have a more advanced myeloma and a shorter survival than patients with ISS stage 1 disease. More recently, the ISS Staging System was revised (R-ISS) to incorporate both chromosomal abnormalities (specifically iFISH), and serum lactate dehydrogenase (LDH), in order to more effectively stratify newly diagnosed myeloma patients based on their survival risk. Chromosomal abnormalities detected by interphase fluorescent in situ hybridization (iFISH) are an important component of defining the biologic characteristics of myeloma. Several studies have demonstrated lower survival outcomes in patients with high-risk disease. LDH is also an important biomarker in multiple myeloma and a level above the upper limit of normal is suggestive of aggressive disease. The R-ISS staging system has been shown to improve prognostic power compared with the individual use of ISS staging, LDH, and cytogenetic abnormalities.***

> **Stage 1** – ISS stage 1 + standard risk chromosomal abnormalities by iFISH + normal LDH
> **Stage 2** – Neither R-ISS stage 1 or/nor 3
> **Stage 3** – ISS stage 3 and either high-risk chromosomal abnormalities by iFISH or high LDH

- High-Risk iFISH – d(17p) and/or t(4;14) and/or t(4;16)
- Standard Risk iFISH – no high-risk chromosomal abnormalities
- High LDH – Serum LDH > upper limit of normal
- Normal LDH – Serum LDH < upper limit of normal

While the ISS and R-ISS staging systems are useful in their ability to allow for comparison of outcomes across clinical trials and stratification of patient disease status to some degree, they have important limitations. These staging systems do not have a prognostic role in early stage myeloma such as MGUS and smoldering MM. Additionally, they do not provide a sufficient estimate of tumor burden and have limited utility for treatment-related risk stratification. Finally, it remains to be seen whether these systems will retain their prognostic significance in the era of novel treatment strategies (see Chapter 4).

***Palumbo A, Avet-Loiseau H, Oliva S, et al. Revised International Staging System for Multiple Myeloma: A Report From International Myeloma Working Group. *J. Clin. Oncol.* 2015;33(26):2863–2869.

TABLE 3-5 Prognostic Factors in Multiple Myeloma

Tumor Biology	Tumor Burden	Patient Related
Ploidy 17p– (p53 deletion) t(14;16) t(14;20) t(4;14) Deletion 13 on conventional cytogenetics Alterations in chromosome 1 t(11;14) t(6;14) LDH levels Plasma cell proliferativerate Presentation as plasma cell leukemia High-risk GEP signature[62]	Durie-Salmon stage International Staging System stage Extramedullary disease	ECOG performance status[63] Age Renal function

ECOG = Eastern Cooperative Oncology Group; GEP = gene expression profile.
Reproduced from Mikhael JR et al. Management of newly diagnosed symptomatic multiple myeloma: Updated Mayo Stratification of Myeloma and Risk-Adapted Therapy (mSMART) Consensus Guidelines 2013. Mayo Clinic Proceedings. 2013;4:360-376. Copyright 2013, with permission from Elsevier.

▶ Prognostic Factors in Multiple Myeloma

Myeloma is a heterogeneous disease and many factors can contribute to the prognosis and the overall outcome. Prognostic factors can be divided into host factors, intrinsic factors, and biochemical markers. The host factors include the age and the performance status of a patient. The intrinsic factors or intrinsic characteristics of the malignant plasma cells include cytogenetic abnormalities and proliferation activity. The biochemical markers reflect the tumor burden and the MM-associated complications. The most commonly recognized prognostic factors for patients with multiple myeloma are summarized in **TABLE 3-5**.

62 GEP signature refers to a single or a combined gene expression change with specificity in terms of prognosis.
63 ECOG performance status is a scale that describes a patient's level of function in terms of physical activity, daily activity, and ability to care for oneself.

TABLE 3-6 Mayo Clinic Stratification of Multiple Myeloma and Risk-Adapted Therapy (mSMART)		
High Risk	**Intermediate Risk**	**Standard Risk**
Any of the following: Deletion 17p t(14;16) by FISH t(14;20) by FISH GEP high-risk signature	t(4;14) by FISH Cytogenetic deletion 13 Plasma cell labeling index[64] >3.0	All other including: t(11;14) by FISH t(6;14) by FISH

Modified from Mikhael JR et al. Management of newly diagnosed symptomatic multiple myeloma: Updated Mayo Stratification of Myeloma and Risk-Adapted Therapy (mSMART) Consensus Guidelines 2013. *Mayo Clinic Proceedings*. 4:360-376. Copyright 2013, with permission from Elsevier.

As listed above, genetic abnormalities are important prognostic factors in MM. Genetic abnormalities observed in myeloma cells is one of the most powerful indicators of tumor aggressiveness. Patients with newly diagnosed multiple myeloma are therefore classified as having high-, intermediate-, or standard-risk disease dependent on their tumor genetics (**TABLE 3-6**).

Patients with standard-risk disease lack high- or intermediate-risk genetic abnormalities. These patients have the best median survival outcomes based on current treatment strategies. Patients with genetic abnormalities indicating high-risk disease tend to have a more aggressive form of myeloma, which may shorten survival. Patients with high-risk disease are often treated in a more aggressive fashion. The intermediate-risk disease category is a classification that was previously considered to be part of the high-risk category. However, with appropriate treatment, patients

---

64 Plasma cell labeling index refers to a measure of plasma cell proliferative activity and functions as a prognostic indicator in newly diagnosed MM.

in this category have been shown to achieve median outcomes similar to that of standard-risk myeloma. The development of new prognostic markers including gene expression profile (GEP) and next-generation sequencing (NGS) are continuously evolving and may soon be incorporated into the risk classification for multiple myeloma. Our ability to effectively optimize and refine prognostic models will eventually lead to enhanced therapeutic approaches and improved patient outcomes.

CHAPTER 4

Response Assessment and Introduction to Treatment

T reatment is indicated for patients with symptoms that fulfill the diagnostic criteria of multiple myeloma including patients with positive biomarkers of malignancy based on the revised IMWG criteria for myeloma: (1) at least 60% clonal plasma cells in the bone marrow, (2) involved/uninvolved serum free light-chain ratio ≥100, and (3) more than one focal lytic lesion detected by MRI greater than or equal to 5 mm in size (see Chapter 3).

Patients with asymptomatic or indolent myeloma are generally monitored every 3 months, with physical examination and measurement of serum and urine M-protein if no myeloma-defining events (MDEs) are present (see Chapter 3). Bone X-rays and bone marrow examinations can be performed less often or when new signs or symptoms occur. The introduction of newer agents may change current treatment guidelines for asymptomatic or indolent myeloma in the near future, particularly for patients harboring features indicative of high-risk disease. For the moment, the consensus is that treatment should be delivered, in most cases, only to patients with symptoms or with radiological evidence of bone disease. Once the treatment has been initiated, patients should be monitored regularly to determine disease status and response to therapy. It is helpful to check the M-protein level after each cycle of treatment, particularly during induction[1] and consolidation,[2] to determine the speed of response. Routine follow-ups with measurement of the serum and urine paraprotein after completion of therapy are necessary to assess the durability of response. Patients with nonsecretory myeloma[3] can be monitored with serial bone marrow aspirations and biopsies. Radiological tests are less helpful to assess response but they can be used to determine if a patient is progressing.

▶ Assessment of Response

Over the past several years, many groups worldwide have proposed and have used different systems to evaluate response to therapy in multiple myeloma (**TABLE 4-1**).

In addition to being complicated, these systems are not comparable to each other. Most importantly of all, they didn't include a definition of complete remission (CR)[4] (see ahead). In the 1990s, with the introduction of high-dose therapy, the number of patients achieving CR increased and it became apparent that there was a strict correlation between CR and improved survival. This correlation, however, was not necessarily true for patients treated with conventional dose chemotherapy. Presumably the level of minimal residual disease after high-dose therapy is lower than after conventional dose chemotherapy. If the CR achieved with the newer antimyeloma agents is comparable to the CR achieved with high-dose therapy remains yet to be determined. Nevertheless, assessing response after high-dose therapy and determining if a patient was in CR became crucial and therefore in 1998, the European Group for Blood and Marrow Transplantation (EBMT), the International

---

1 Induction therapy refers to the initial treatment used to bring a newly diagnosed patient's disease into remission.

2 Consolidation refers to treatment, such as a stem cell transplant, given after the initial therapy to decrease a patient's disease state to a greater extent.

3 Nonsecretory myeloma is a rare variant of multiple myeloma in which no monoclonal protein (M-spike) is produced, making diagnosis and disease staging difficult. The clinical presentation and radiographic findings are identical to that of multiple myeloma.

4 Complete remission (CR) refers to the disappearance of all, or nearly all, detectable signs of cancer in response to treatment.

TABLE 4-1 Criteria to Define Response in Multiple Myeloma

Myeloma Task Force	Southwest Oncology Group	Medical Research Council
1. Reduction of M-protein to 50% or less from initial baseline value 2. Reduction of light-chain excretion in the urine to 50% or less from initial baseline value 3. Reduction of 50% in size of plasmacytomas 4. Radiological evidence of skeletal healing *One or more of the above criteria required	1. Reduction of calculated synthetic serum protein to 25% or less from initial baseline value 2. Reduction of urine light-chain excretion to less than 10% or less than 0.2 g/24 hours of initial baseline value 3. Improvement in bone pain and performance status 4. Correction of anemia and low albumin if due to MM *All the above criteria sustained for at least 2 months	1. Stable or nondetectable M-protein for at least 3 months 2. Stable or nondetectable urine light-chain excretion for at least 3 months 3. Few or no MM-associated symptoms 4. No transfusion requirement *All criteria above required

Data from Kyle R, Rajkumar S. Criteria for diagnosis, staging, risk stratification and response assessment of multiple myeloma. *Leukemia.* 2009;23(1):3-9.

Bone Marrow Transplant Registry (IBMTR), and the Autologous Blood and Marrow Transplant Registry (ABMTR) with Dr. Bladé as the leading author, published criteria for response in patients with multiple myeloma (**TABLE 4-2**). The EBMT/IBMTR/ABMTR criteria

TABLE 4-2 EBMT, IBMTR, and ABMTR Criteria for Response, Relapse, and Progression in Patients with Multiple Myeloma

Response to Treatment	Definition
Complete response (CR)	Requires all of the following: 1. Absence of the M-protein by IFE (immunofixation) maintained for at least 6 weeks 2. <5% plasma cells in a bone marrow aspirate or biopsy 3. No new lytic lesions or increase in the size of old lesions on skeletal X-rays 4. Disappearance of soft tissue plasmacytomas
Partial response (PR)	Requires all of the following: 1. >50% reduction in the serum M-protein maintained for at least 6 weeks 2. Reduction of 24 hours urine light-chain protein either by >90% or to <200 mg maintained for at least 6 weeks 3. For patients with nonsecretory MM only, >50% reduction in plasma cells in a bone marrow aspirate and biopsy, maintained for at least 6 weeks 4. >50% reduction in size of soft-tissue plasmacytomas 5. No new lytic lesions or increase in the size of old lesions on skeletal X-rays
Minimal response (MR)	Requires all of the following: 1. 25%–49% reduction in the serum M-protein maintained for at least 6 weeks 2. 50%–89% reduction of 24 hours urine light-chain protein maintained for at least 6 weeks 3. For patients with nonsecretory MM only, 25%–49% reduction in plasma cells in a bone marrow aspirate and biopsy, maintained for at least 6 weeks 4. 25%–49% reduction in size of soft-tissue plasmacytomas 5. No new lytic lesions or increase in the size of old lesions on skeletal X-rays

(continues)

TABLE 4-2 EBMT, IBMTR, and ABMTR Criteria for Response, Relapse, and Progression in Patients with Multiple Myeloma (*Continued*)

Response to Treatment	Definition
No change (NC)	1. Not meeting the criteria of either minimal response or progressive disease
Relapse from CR	Requires at least one of the following: 1. Reappearance of serum or urine M-protein on IFE or electrophoresis, confirmed by at least one further investigation and excluding oligoclonal reconstitution[5] 2. >5% plasma cells in a bone marrow aspirate or biopsy 3. Development of new lytic bone lesions or soft-tissue plasmacytomas or increase in size of residual bone lesions 4. Development of hypercalcemia
Progressive disease for patients not in CR	Requires at least one of the following: 1. >25% increase in the level of serum M-protein, confirmed by at least one repeat observation 2. >25% increase in 24-hours urine light-chain protein, confirmed by at least one repeat observation 3. >25% plasma cells in a bone marrow aspirate or biopsy 4. Development of new lytic bone lesions or soft-tissue plasmacytomas or increase in size of residual bone lesions or soft tissue plasmacytomas 5. Development of hypercalcemia

Criteria for evaluating disease response and progression in patients with multiple myeloma treated by high-dose therapy and haemopoietic stem cell transplantation. Myeloma Subcommittee of the EBMT. European Group for Blood and Marrow Transplant. *Br J Haematol.* 1998;5:1115-1123.

---

5 Oligoclonal reconstitution is the representation of a reconstituting immune system via faint bands appearing on an immunofixation result, generally after transplant. This phenomenon can be present for several months and often resolves spontaneously.

include a more accurate definition of complete remission, as well as a definition of relapse from complete remission and a definition of progression.

These criteria, also known as the Bladé criteria, were initially proposed to assess only patients after high-dose therapy and stem cell rescue, but subsequently they started to be used to assess response in stages of treatment.

The major limitations of the Bladé criteria are the lack of a precise and stringent definition of CR and the lack of the incorporation of the free light chain assay to determine response in patients with oligosecretory myeloma.[6] With the introduction of the new anti-MM agents, it became clear that it was important to use more reproducible criteria to allow a fair comparison between strategies and to assess the quality of the response. To overcome these problems the International Multiple Myeloma Working Group lead by Dr. Brian Durie, revised and published in 2006, the new international uniform response criteria for multiple myeloma (**TABLE 4-3**).

The most important changes in the current criteria compared to the older systems are the introduction of two newer response categories: the stringent complete remission (sCR) and the very good partial response (VGPR). The newer uniform criteria also include the free light chain assay for interpreting response in patients with nondetectable M-protein by standard electrophoresis. The criteria for defining progressive disease and relapse from CR remain unchanged, however a new category for clinical relapse was added. This category was established to emphasize that early retreatment is unnecessary until patients become symptomatic, to avoid occurrence of unwanted toxicity. The uniform criteria are widely used to evaluate response to therapy in clinical trials.

As described in Chapter 3, assessment of minimal residual disease (MRD) is becoming an increasingly important modality by which to assess deep levels of disease response to treatment. The introduction of highly efficacious therapies has led to a dramatic increase in the number of patients that achieve a complete remission (CR). In this

---

6 Oligosecretory myeloma is a form of myeloma in which the myeloma cells produce much less protein relative to the quantity of malignant cells in the bone marrow.

TABLE 4-3 International Myeloma Working Group Uniform Response Criteria

Response to Treatment	Definition
Stringent complete remission (sCR)	Normal free light chain ratio and absence of maliganant plasma cell in the bone marrow
Complete remission (CR)	1. <5% maliganant plasma cells in bone marrow 2. Negative immunofixation on serum and urine electrophoresis tests 3. Disappearance of any soft-tissue plasmacytomas
Very good partial response (VGPR)	1. Serum and urine detected by immunofixation but not by electrophoresis or 2. >90% reduction in serum M-protein plus urine M-protein level <l00 mg/24 hours
Partial response (PR)	1. >50% reduction of serum M-protein and reduction of urine M-protein by >90% or to <200 mg per 24 hrs 2. If serum and urine M-protein are non-detectable by electrophoresis, a >50% reduction of free light chain levels is required 3. *For patients with nonsecretory disease* >50% reduction in plasma cells is required in place of M-protein (bone marrow at baseline needs to have >30% infiltration) 4. If present at baseline a >50% reduction in the size of soft-tissue plasmacytoma is also required
Stable disease (SD)	1. Not meeting the criteria for CR, VGPR, PR, or progression

(continues)

TABLE 4-3 International Myeloma Working Group Uniform Response Criteria (*Continued*)

Response to Treatment	Definition
Progressive disease (PD)	Requires any one or more of the following. Increase of >25% from baseline in: 1. Serum M-protein (absolute >0.5 g/dL) 2. Urine M-protein (absolute >200 mg/24 hrs) 3. In patients with otherwise not measurable disease, increase of >10 mg/dL between involved and uninvolved FLC levels 4. Bone marrow plasma cell percentage (absolute >10%) 5. Development of new bone lesions or soft-tissue plasmacytomas or increase in the size of existing bone lesions or soft-tissue plasmacytomas 6. Development of hypercalcemia (due to MM)
Clinical relapse	Require one or more of: 1. Development of new soft-tissue plasmacytomas or bone lesions 2. Increase in size of existing soft-tissue plasmacytomas or bone lesions 3. Hypercalcemia 4. Decrease in Hgb of >2 g/dL 5. Rise in serum creatinine by >2 mg/dL
Relapse from CR	Require any one or more of the following: 1. Reappearance of serum or urine M-protein by SPEP, UPEP, and IFE 2. Development of >5% plasma cells in the bone marrow 3. Appearance of any other sign of progression (new plasmacytomas, lytic bone lesion, or hypercalcemia)

context, MRD can be used to push deeper and evaluate the true quality of response achieved. Recent studies have suggested that patients capable of achieving a deep MRD-negative response may have improved progression-free and long-term survival. Additionally, information from MRD testing can in the future help inform treatment decisions. For example, a physician treating a patient with high-risk disease that has achieved a CR but is MRD-positive may wish to refrain from stopping treatment. MRD is increasingly becoming implemented across clinical trials and several academic institutions started to use it more regularly to assess patient responses. In 2016, the IMWG updated the criteria of response adding MRD testing as a measurement of depth of response (**TABLE 4-4**). In 2017, the NCCN (National Cancer Comprehensive Network) guidelines recommended MRD testing for measurement of depth of response.

TABLE 4-4 IMWG Criteria for Response and Assessment in Multiple Myeloma	
Treatment Response	**Criteria**
Sustained MRD-negative	MRD negative in the marrow and by imaging confirmed minimum of 1 year apart
Flow MRD-negative	Absence of phenotypically abnormal plasma cells by NGF on bone marrow, using EuroFlow standard operation procedure with a minimum sensitivity of 1 in 105 nucleated cells or higher
Sequencing MRD-negative	Absence of phenotypically abnormal plasma cells by NGS on bone marrow, using LymphoSIGHT platform (or equivalent validated method) with a minimum sensitivity of 1 in 105 nucleated cells or higher
Imaging plus MRD-negative	MRD negativity by NGF or NGS plus negative PET/CT

NGF = next-generation flow; NGS = next-generation sequencing.
Data from Kumar, S. et al. (2017). Multiple Myeloma, Version 3. 2017, NCCN Clinical Practice Guidelines in Oncology. Journal of the National Comprehensive Cancer Network, 15(2), 230–269

▶ Clinical Trials

Before discussing treatment options for MM, it is important to discuss the role of clinical trials because all available treatments for myeloma are first tested in these studies. There are many different types of trials, but the most convincing evidence that a treatment is superior to others comes from large prospective randomized clinical trials.

A randomized study is a clinical trial in which all patients are randomly (as if a coin were flipped) assigned to receive a particular treatment. The likelihood of receiving one or the other treatment is identical. The results of such studies are thought to be more reliable than studies that are not randomized because there is less chance that study will be biased. In a prospective study patients are chosen before treatment and observed during the period of treatment. In these studies, the type of patients to be studied and the information collected is decided upon before the study begins, so it is less biased than a retrospective study.

A retrospective study is conducted by reviewing patient medical records to see if groups of patients that had different treatments had different outcomes. If the only difference between the groups was their treatment, then the different outcome presumably resulted from the treatment. A phase I clinical trial is a study designed to determine if a new drug is safe. Usually a phase I clinical trial is a small study involving only few patients. A phase II clinical trial intends to evaluate the efficacy of a treatment for a specific condition and possible side effects are monitored. A phase III is a large clinical trial designed to evaluate a drug that demonstrated promising activity with tolerable side effects in phase I and phase II studies. After successful conclusion of a phase III clinical trial, the drug or combination of drugs may receive formal approval from the US Food and Drug Administration (FDA) to be sold as a licensed drug if the drug appears to have acceptable side effects and activity against the specific disease.

One of the biggest challenges in treating multiple myeloma over the last decade is that new promising treatment regimens are constantly being developed. Some of the new regimens that look promising in Phase II trials have not completed the lengthy testing needed for the more convincing randomized Phase III trials. In addition, there are now so many potential combinations of treatments for myeloma that comparing them all to each other is not always feasible.

Lastly, even Phase III trials themselves can be less than convincing because of how the study was conducted or alternatively, in the time it took to conduct and analyze a study, new promising treatments may have been identified that make the prior study already out of date. In the second part of this chapter, we will discuss a variety of treatment options as well as the current evidence to support their use in the treatment of MM.

▶ Chemotherapy

Chemotherapy is the broad term used for any treatment involving the use of drugs that stop the growth of cancer cells. Chemotherapy is generally considered a systemic treatment because it can attack cancer cells throughout the body. Chemotherapy can be administered through a vein, taken by mouth, or can be injected directly into the tumor or a body cavity. While chemotherapy works by killing fast-growing cancer cells, unfortunately, it also kills other fast-growing cells in the body including hair, blood cells, and cells of the gastrointestinal tract. The most common side effects of chemotherapy are nausea, vomiting, diarrhea, hair loss, and marrow suppression. Chemotherapy can also cause organ damage such as kidney, lung, liver, and cardiac toxicity.

Different chemotherapy drugs may target specific types of cancer cells. For example, alkylating agents[7] are a commonly used type of chemotherapy treatment for myeloma. Their mechanism of action is to damage the DNA inside cancer cells, thus preventing proliferation of the malignant cells. A chemotherapy regimen usually includes a combination of drugs that work together to attack the same type of cancer cells but with different attack sites. Normally a chemotherapy regimen is given to patients in cycles, where each cycle consists of a short period of treatment followed by a period of rest. Chemotherapy administered in cycles is more effective at killing tumor cells that are dividing rapidly. Also, during the rest period patients can recover from the side effects induced by the chemotherapy drugs.

---

7 Alkylating agents are chemotherapeutic agents that work against myeloma cells by cross-linking DNA and blocking cell division.

TABLE 4-5 Chemotherapy Drugs Active Against Myeloma Cells	
Drug	**Administration**
Melphalan	Oral or vein
Cyclophosphamide	Oral or vein
Carmustine (BCNU)	Vein
Cytarabine (Ara-C)	Vein
Etoposide	Oral or vein
Cisplatin	Vein
Vincristine	Vein
Adryamicin (doxorubicin)	Vein
Doxil (pegylated-doxorubicin)	Vein
Bendamustine	Vein

Chemotherapy can be administered in standard or conventional dose or can be given in high dose prior to stem cell transplant. The most common FDA-approved chemotherapy drugs used alone or in combination to treat myeloma are listed in **TABLE 4-5**.

Bendamustine (Treanda©)

Bendamustine is a chemotherapy drug, specifically an alkylating agent that has been approved in Germany for several years to treat certain cancers including myeloma. Through its function as an alkylating agent, bendamustine damages the DNA of myeloma cells beyond repair, resulting in their death. While bendamustine is currently approved by the FDA in the US for the treatment of two blood cancers, it has yet to be approved for use in myeloma outside of a clinical trial.

Phase I/II studies investigating bendamustine in combination with lenalidomide and dexamethasone illustrated an overall response rate of greater than 50% in relapsed or refractory patients. Additionally, a phase II study investigating bendamustine in combination with bortezomib and dexamethasone reported a response rate of 68% in patients who had received one or more prior therapies. In a phase III study involving the use combination of bendamustine and prednisone compared against melphalan and prednisone for newly diagnosed patients, therapy with bendamustine-prednisone presented a higher overall response rate and a 19% higher complete response (CR) rate.

Bendamustine is given intravenously over an infusion lasting 30 minutes to an hour, and the optimal dosage has been determined as 60 mg/m^2 when used in combination with thalidomide and dexamethasone (see ahead) for patients with relapsed disease. Commonly reported side effects include low blood cell counts, fever, nausea, and vomiting. These side effects generally cease when the treatment period has ended. More recently bendamustine has been used in combination with lenalidomide, pomalidomide, and ixazomib showing excellent response rate in the relapse setting. Current and future studies evaluating the efficacy of bendamustine in relapsed patients, as well as in combination with other drugs, may serve to provide rationale for its use as an FDA-approved therapy for MM.

▶ Steroids

Corticosteroids are drugs closely related to cortisol, a hormone naturally produced in the adrenal glands. Corticosteroids induce apoptosis[8] of lymphoid cells[9] including plasma cells in culture,[10] while sparing myeloid-derived cells,[11] Patients on steroids have an increased risk

---

8 Apoptosis is a process of programmed cell death.
9 Lymphoid cells refer to a group of blood cells responsible for the production of immunity mediated by cells or antibodies and including lymphocytes, lymphoblasts, and plasma cells.
10 Culture refers to the growth of cells in an artificial environment which have been removed from a living organism.
11 Myeloid-derived cells are a group of cells that belong to the myeloid lineage of blood cells, a family distinct from that of the lymphoid lineage.

of developing infections due to the immunosuppressive nature of the drug. Patients with diabetes may have problems controlling blood sugar levels and some patients may develop new-onset diabetes while receiving steroids. Other common side effects of high-dose steroids are high blood pressure and fluid retention.[12] Psychiatric problems such as mood disorders, anxiety, hallucinations, and insomnia are also quite common particularly in the elderly patients. Steroids can be given alone or in combination with chemotherapy drugs. They can be administered in a vein or taken by mouth. The most common corticosteroids used in myeloma are prednisone and dexamethasone.

The addition of steroids to chemotherapy regimens and to the newer anti-MM agents can increase the response rate without causing the myelosuppression[13] commonly seen with chemotherapy drugs. In 1969, Alexanian and his colleagues compared oral melphalan to melphalan and prednisone for treatment of newly diagnosed MM. The addition of prednisone not only increased the response rate but also improved the survival of patients. Subsequently, the addition of steroids to chemotherapy regimens became the standard of care. When administered at high dose, steroids alone can produce rapid response both in newly diagnosed patients and in patients with relapsed MM. Approximately 40% of newly diagnosed patients and 25% of relapsed patients will respond to single-agent high-dose dexamethasone. High-dose dexamethasone given alone or as part of a chemotherapy regimen is generally administered in "pulse doses"[14] (40 mg every day for 4 days, followed by 4 days off, per 3 times every month). Because steroids toxicity increases exponentially with the dose of administration, some of the newer clinical trials are designed to explore different and less toxic doses of dexamethasone combined to other effective antimyeloma agents.

---

12 Fluid retention refers to excess fluid that collects in the tissues of the body, commonly identified by swelling in the feet and lower legs.
13 Myelosuppression is a decrease in the production of red blood cells, platelets, and certain white blood cells as a result of diminished bone marrow activity.
14 Pulse doses are characterized by the administration of large doses of a medication in an intermittent manner to reduce side effects and enhance therapeutic effects.

▶ Interferon-α

Interferons (IFN) are proteins naturally produced in the body by the cells of the immune system—leukocytes,[15] fibroblasts,[16] and T-lymphocytes. IFN is produced in small quantity in response to antigens such as viruses, bacteria, or tumor cells. Interferon can be used to treat some types of cancer, including myeloma. However, the number of patients with myeloma that respond to IFN alone is too low to justify toxicity and cost. For example, in 2001 the Myeloma Trialist Collaborative Group published a large meta-analysis[17] of 24 trials involving more than 4000 patients with myeloma treated with interferon. While the response and the response duration were slightly better in the IFN group, there was no difference in survival between the two groups.

Usually, IFN is given following a prior chemotherapy regimen as maintenance to keep the myeloma from returning. In the maintenance setting, the addition of IFN has been shown to prolong progression-free survival[18] but not overall survival,[19] suggesting that patients receiving IFN may develop a more resistant myeloma. The two main recombinant types of IFN used clinically are α and γ. Interferon is administered as an injection subcutaneously (under the skin), usually in the thigh or abdomen, and it is generally given 3 days a week. The most common dose is 3 MU/m²

---

15 Leukocyte is another term for a white blood cell (WBC).
16 Fibroblasts are cells in the connective tissues that generate the structural framework for animal tissues.
17 Meta-analysis is a statistical technique combining results from multiple independent studies in order to assess the clinical effectiveness of a particular treatment or procedure.
18 Progression-free survival (PFS) refers to the time period in which the patient survives before the myeloma progresses or relapses. It is the improved survival of a patient that is directly correlated to the effectiveness of the myeloma treatment. When expressed in the context of a clinical trial, this term reflects the median-PFS for all patients, though the notation often remains as "PFS".
19 Overall survival (OS) refers to the time period between initiation of therapy and death. When expressed in the context of a clinical trial, this term reflects the median-OS for all patients, though the notation often remains as "OS".

given three times per week. Interferon works against myeloma in different ways, directly attacking the cancer cells and indirectly strengthening the body's immune system.

Common side effects of IFN are fatigue, flu-like symptoms (fever, chills, muscle and joint pain), nausea, vomiting, and lack of appetite. Patients taking IFN can experience skin irritation at the site of injection, dizziness, and peripheral neuropathy (tingling and abnormal sensation of hands and toes). Less commonly, it can cause hypothyroidism,[20] ocular side effects,[21] arrhythmias,[22] diarrhea, and liver abnormalities. IFN may also suppress the production of white blood cells, red blood cells, and platelets, and it can cause infertility. Because two-thirds of patients taking IFN will experience some side effects and its activity against myeloma is not very high, this drug is seldom used in the United States.

▶ Arsenic Trioxide

In the mid 1990s, two research groups in China reported that arsenic is an effective and safe treatment for patients with a type of acute leukemia also known as acute promyelocytic leukemia. Subsequently, these findings have been confirmed in the United States and currently arsenic is approved for the treatment of patients with relapsed or refractory acute promyelocytic leukemia. Arsenic has been shown promise in the treatment of other malignancies including multiple myeloma.

Arsenic works in vitro against MM by inhibiting both the JAK/STAT3 and nuclear factor (NF)-κB signaling pathways, by decreasing the production of IL-6, and by inducing apoptosis in both drug-sensitive and resistant MM cell lines. It also upregulates the expression of TRAIL (tumor necrosis factor-related apoptosis inducing ligand receptors).[23] Arsenic has been evaluated in clinical trials as

---

20 Hypothyroidism is a condition in which the body lacks sufficient thyroid hormone.
21 Ocular side effects are side effects associated with the eyes or vision.
22 Arrhythmia refers to an abnormal beating of the heart, which is often times harmless but can be life threatening in some cases.
23 TRAIL is a cytokine protein that functions to induce cellular apoptosis.

a single agent and in combination with other agents. For example, ascorbic acid can potentiate the effects of arsenic by reducing glutathione[24] inside the cells. Intracellular glutathione is important for repairing mithocondrial damage.[25] Arsenic has also been evaluated in combination with dexamethasone, bortezomib, and melphalan and currently numerous trials are underway to confirm its activity against MM. Arsenic is administered intravenously over 1 to 2 hours. The recommended dose of arsenic is 0.25 mg/kg/day for 5 days/ week for 2 weeks followed by 2 weeks of rest, or it can be given at the dose of 0.25 mg/kg/day twice a week.

The most common side effects of arsenic include nausea, vomiting, diarrhea or constipation, abdominal pain, fatigue, weakness, headache, peripheral edema, rash, itching, sore throat, and cough. Arsenic should not be given to patients with history of arrhythmia or heart failure or to patients with renal insufficiency. The significant toxicities associated with this drug prevent its widespread clinical use.

▶ Radiotherapy

Radiotherapy means using a certain type of energy called *ionizing radiation* to treat cancer. The radiation used is similar to that used for X-rays but it is given at a much higher dose. Radiation therapy destroys the malignant cells in the area being treated (the target tissue) by damaging their genetic material, making it impossible for these cells to continue to grow. Radiation therapy can also damage the normal cells in the surrounding tissues, however, most normal cells can recover from the effect of radiation therapy. Radiation therapy can cause fatigue and loss of appetite. The skin above the treated area can become irritated similar to bad sunburn. Side effects vary with the total dose, the number and size of fractions,[26] and the area

---

24 Glutathione is an important antioxidant in several classes of organisms including animals.
25 Mitochondrial damage is an injury to the mitochondria, which are structures in our cells that produce energy.
26 Fractions refer to the components (fractions) into which the total radiation dose is divided.

of the body to be treated. Myeloma cells are highly radiosensitive[27] and radiotherapy has been used in the management of myeloma for decades. The main indications for radiotherapy in MM are prevention of further bone destruction, prevention of pathologic fractures, treatment or prevention of nerve-root or spinal cord compression, and controlling pain caused by a bone lesion or by a soft-tissue plasmacytoma. This type of radiation therapy or local radiotherapy is administered in an outpatient basis and it is given at the dose of 1.8–2 Gray (Gy) [28] per fraction, administered once daily, five times a week. The total dose and number of treatments may vary based on the location to treat and the performance status (level of general well being) of the patient. The dose administered is generally lower for pain control (20–25 Gy) and higher to treat spinal cord compression (30–40 Gy) or to control a plasmacytoma (40–45 Gy). Radiotherapy is also recommended following fixation of a pathologic fracture to decrease the risk of further bone destruction. Patients with myeloma may also receive radiation therapy at higher doses to the entire body in preparation for stem cell transplant (see Chapter 5), termed total body irradiation (TBI). A randomized study comparing melphalan-TBI to melphalan alone as a conditioning regimen prior to autologous transplant[29] in MM found melphalan-TBI to be inferior to melphalan alone. Because of that, melphalan alone remains the preferred conditioning regimen prior to autologous transplant in MM. TBI is still used to prepare patients for allogeneic transplants.[30] TBI is generally given in fractionated doses twice or three times a day for a total dose of 10–15 Gy.

The most common acute side effects include fatigue, nausea, vomiting, parotiditis,[31] oral mucositis,[32] and skin changes. Late toxicities

---

27 Radiosensitive refers to the condition of cells, tissues, organs, or organisms being readily affected by radiation.
28 Gray (Gy) is a unit used to measure the dose of ionizing radiation.
29 Autologous transplant is a type of stem cell transplant that uses the individual's own stem cells.
30 Allogeneic transplant is a type of stem cell transplant in which the patient receives stem cells from another person.
31 Parotiditis refers to inflammation of the parotid gland.
32 Oral mucositis refers to the breakdown of the cells lining the inside of the mouth, leaving the area vulnerable to ulcers and infection.

can include interstitial pneumonitis,[33] cataracts,[34] hypothyroidism, decreased gonadal[35] function, and liver and kidney damage.

▶ Immunomodulatory Agents

Immunomodulatory agents refer to a class of drugs that are functional and structural analogs of thalidomide (see ahead). While their mechanisms of action have not been fully elucidated, they appear to function against myeloma in two major ways. First, they serve to both activate and enhance immune system cells to attack myeloma cells. Second, they have been shown to function to directly kill myeloma cells through stimulating myeloma cell apoptosis (programmed cell death) via the release of various enzymes[36] in the body, turning on tumor suppressor genes, and activating cytokines that prevent myeloma cell proliferation. The immunomodulatory drugs that are currently used in myeloma treatment are summarized below.

Thalidomide (Thalomid©)

In the late 1950s and early 1960s, thalidomide was marketed outside of the United States for treatment of insomnia. Thalidomide was sold in at least 46 countries under many different brand names. It was used as a sleeping pill, and to treat morning sickness during pregnancy. Because of its association with tragic birth malformations (phocomelia), thalidomide was withdrawn from the market in Germany and United Kingdom in December of 1961. In the mid 1960s, scientists determined that thalidomide was an effective treatment for the skin lesions caused by leprosy. The FDA approved thalidomide for this use only in 1998, more than 30 years later.

In the meantime, researchers continued to investigate the use of this agent to treat a variety of other diseases and conditions, such as

---

33 Pneumonitis is a disease in which the tissue surrounding the small air sacs within the lungs becomes inflamed.
34 Cataracts are characterized by clouding of the normally clear lens of the eye.
35 Gonads are the sex glands of the testes in males and ovaries in females.
36 Enzymes are proteins that increase the rate at which chemical reactions occur.

arthritis, Crohn's disease, HIV-related ulcers, and cancers. One of the main anticancer mechanisms of thalidomide is its prevention of blood vessel formation [by blocking basic fibroblast growth factor and vascular endothelial growth factor (VEGF)]. Blood vessels are necessary to feed the tumor cells. The formation of new blood vessels is a process called angiogenesis. The observations that patients with advanced myeloma have increased angiogenesis in the bone marrow led to the initiation of the first clinical trial of thalidomide at the University of Arkansas. In this pilot trial, one out of five patients with advanced and resistant multiple myeloma achieved a near-complete remission. These results prompted the initiation of a phase II trial of thalidomide for relapsed or refractory MM. All patients enrolled in this trial had previously received and failed many other treatments, including high-dose therapy and stem cell transplant, and approximately 25% of patients responded to thalidomide alone. Since then, several other studies have confirmed the efficacy of thalidomide in MM.

Inhibition of angiogenesis is not the only therapeutic effect of thalidomide. Thalidomide has been shown to directly attack myeloma cells and bone marrow stromal cells by altering the expression of adhesion molecules located on the surface of the tumor cells. Thalidomide also works by stopping the production or altering the function of many cytokines involved in maintaining the myeloma cells, like TNF. Thalidomide is also an immunomodulatory agent and it promotes the growth of anti-CD3 T cells[37] that can inhibit MM cell growth by increasing the level of interferon-α or IL-12. Thalidomide and its analogues directly induce apoptosis (programmed cell death) of plasma cells in culture.

Given its activity as a single agent, thalidomide was then tested in combination with steroids and other chemotherapy drugs active against myeloma. The proportion of patients who respond to thalidomide given in combination with steroids and or chemotherapy is twice as high as the proportion that responded to thalidomide alone. In May of 2006, the FDA approved the use of thalidomide in combination with dexamethasone for the treatment of patients with newly diagnosed multiple myeloma.

---

37 Anti-CD3 T-cells are T cells that are activated via anti-CD3 agents. CD3 refers to a protein cofactor that helps activate cytotoxic T cells.

Thalidomide is taken orally. An intravenous preparation is currently not available because thalidomide is not soluble in water. The drug pharmacokinetics varies among patients. The recommended dose for newly diagnosed patients is 200 mg a day. However, some studies have reported responses at doses of 100 mg or less/day. The maximum concentration is reached within 4 hours and the half-life in the blood is longer when thalidomide is given at higher doses. The absorbed drug is metabolized in the liver and its metabolites are rapidly excreted in urine, while unabsorbed drug is excreted in the feces. Thalidomide is well tolerated in patients with renal insufficiency at moderate doses, while the appropriate dose for patients with liver failure has not been yet determined. Thalidomide is teratogenic[38] and therefore is absolutely contraindicated in pregnant women.

Thalidomide is available only by prescription from physicians and pharmacies registered in the System for Thalidomide Education and Prescribing Safety (S.T.E.P.S.) program. The S.T.E.P.S. program is a restricted distribution program designed to prevent fetal exposure. The program involves:

- Required pregnancy testing
- Required birth control measures
- Physician education
- Patient education
- Registration
- Patient informed consent forms

Women of childbearing potential are required to take a pregnancy test every month and they are required to be on two effective forms of birth control. Men receiving thalidomide who are sexually active must use a latex condom.

The most common side effects observed with thalidomide are fatigue, sedation, dizziness, constipation, dry mouth, and dry skin. A peripheral neuropathy (decreased sensation associated with burning and tingling) of hands and feet is a problem particularly after prolonged exposure. In some patients, thalidomide may also suppress the production of the white blood cells. The toxicity of

---

38 Teratogenic refers to any agent that disturbs the development of a fetus or embryo.

thalidomide appears to be dose related. In general these side effects can be controlled with dose adjustment. Most side effects, but not the peripheral neuropathy, are reversible, and they subside after stopping the drug. Because sedation[39] is a frequent side effect, thalidomide should be taken at bedtime. Occasionally, patients may develop an erythematous macular papular skin rash.[40] The rash is generally self limiting, but thalidomide should be stopped until clearing of the rash and then restarted at a lower dose. Very rarely, cases of Steven-Johnson syndrome[41] have been reported. Other less common side effects observed in patients taking thalidomide are hypothyroidism, peripheral edema,[42] tremors,[43] and bradycardia.[44] One of the most serious side effects of thalidomide, when given in combination with steroids or a steroid anthracycline[45] combination, is the development of a thrombotic event or deep vein thrombosis (DVT).[46] The incidence is approximately 15%. DVT is a condition where a blood clot forms in one of the deep veins, usually in the legs or abdomen. Patient will experience swelling, pain, and redness at the site of the blood clot. When a small piece of clot detaches from the leg and travels to the lung it causes a serious and at times deadly condition called pulmonary embolism.[47] Therapeutic anticoagulation [warfarin (Coumadin) and/or enoxaparin (Lovenox)] should be used

---

39 Sedation is the state of calm or sleep produced by the administration of a particular drug.

40 Erythematous macular papular skin rash is a type of rash characterized by a flat, red area on the skin covered with small, elevated bumps.

41 Steven-Johnson syndrome is a disorder of the skin and mucous membranes characterized by flu-like symptoms and a painful rash.

42 Peripheral edema refers to the accumulation fluid and subsequent swelling of tissues supplied by the peripheral vascular system (often the legs and/or arms).

43 Tremors are an abnormal and repetitive shaking movement of the body.

44 Bradycardia refers to a slower than normal heart rate, generally lower than 60 beats per minute.

45 Anthracyclines are a class of chemotherapy drugs used in the treatment of cancer.

46 Deep vein thrombosis (DVT) is a condition that occurs when a blood clot forms in one or more deep veins in the body, most commonly the legs.

47 Pulmonary embolism is a sudden blockage of a major artery in the lung due to a blood clot.

in patients receiving thalidomide in combination with steroids or a steroid-anthracycline combination, and in patients with other risk factors for thrombosis.[48]

Lenalidomide (Revlimid©)

Lenalidomide is a member of a newer class of novel immunomodulatory drug (IMiD) analogues of thalidomide. These drugs are structurally very similar to thalidomide but are more potent and have a different side effect profile than thalidomide. Like thalidomide, lenalidomide has many mechanisms of anti-MM activity. Lenalidomide directly induces apoptosis of multiple myeloma cells, inhibits tumor-associated angiogenesis, augments natural killer cell (NK) activity against MM cells, and downregulates NF-κB.[49] Lenalidomide also works by altering the function or blocking the production of numerous key growth factors in MM (such as IL-6) and by inhibiting adhesion of MM cells to bone marrow stromal cells.

Based on its promising anti-MM activity in vitro, the first phase I clinical trial of lenalidomide in MM was conducted and then published in 2002. In that study, 25 patients with relapsed, refractory MM received lenalidomide as a single agent. Anti-MM activity was observed in approximately one-third of the patients and the main side effect observed was reversible myelosuppression. In a subsequent phase II study, patients who failed to respond to lenalidomide as a single agent achieved a response with the addition of dexamethasone, providing the rationale for the use of lenalidomide in combination with steroids or with other anti-MM agents. Shortly after, two large studies aimed to evaluate the effect of lenalidomide combined with dexamethasone versus dexamethasone alone in patients with relapsed or refractory MM were initiated simultaneously in the United States and in Europe. Both studies showed that patients treated with the lenalidomide-dexamethasone combination had better outcomes; rates of response and duration of responses were significantly higher. Based on the positive results of these two studies, in 2006 the FDA approved lenalidomide in combination with dexamethasone as

---

48 Thrombosis refers to clotting of the blood in part of the circulatory system.

49 NF-κB is a protein complex that controls gene expression, cell survival, and cytokine expression.

treatment for patients with myeloma who have received at least one prior therapy. Lenalidomide in combination with dexamethasone and with other anti-MM agents is currently used in patients with newly diagnosed as well as relapsed myeloma.

Lenalidomide is administered orally and the recommended dose is 25 mg daily on days 1 to 21 of every 28 days. Lenalidomide is eliminated via the kidney and therefore the dose needs to be adjusted in patients with kidney impairment. The drug should be taken with water. Lenalidomide doesn't appear to have the teratogenic effect of thalidomide; however, the real risk of birth defect is still unknown and therefore precautions should be taken to avoid pregnancy. To prevent exposure during pregnancy a risk-management plan called RevAssist has been implemented. Only physicians or pharmacists registered with RevAssist can prescribe and dispense the drug.

The most common side effect of lenalidomide is myelosuppression occurring in more than half of previously treated patients and in approximately one-third of previously untreated patients. It is recommended to check blood count every week or every other week during the first 2 months of treatment with lenalidomide and on a monthly basis thereafter. The dose of lenalidomide should be adjusted appropriately when and if the number of platelets and/or white cells falls to a low and unsafe level. Like thalidomide, lenalidomide can cause thromboembolic events. The incidence of thrombotic events appears to be higher in patients taking concomitant dexamethasone, erythropoietin, or darbepoietin (see Chapter 7). Aspirin prophylaxis has been used successfully for prevention of thrombotic events, despite their venous (of the vein) origin, in patients receiving lenalidomide. However, therapeutic anti-coagulation is strongly recommended in patients receiving lenalidomide in combination with high-dose steroids or a steroid-anthracycline combination, and in patients with other risk factors for thrombosis. Other side effects of lenalidomide include fatigue, muscle cramps, nausea, decreased appetite, diarrhea or constipation, dizziness, anxiety, elevation of liver enzymes, and occasionally a self-limiting rash. Less commonly it can cause inflammation of the lungs, a complication called pneumonitis, presenting with shortness of breath and fatigue requiring discontinuation of treatment. Peripheral neuropathy is much less frequent than with thalidomide, occurring in $<10\%$ of patients.

In 2017, the FDA approved low-dose lenalidomide (~10 mg) in the maintenance setting, after autologous transplant or after induction therapy, based on the results of several large randomized studies showing that lenalidomide maintenance can prolong the duration of response and life expectancy of patients with MM.

Pomalidomide (Pomalyst©)

Pomalidomide, like lenalidomide, is another derivative or analog of thalidomide but with more potent immunosuppression activity, and is used in the treatment of relapsed and refractory myeloma. Pomalidomide works both directly against myeloma cells as well as their support systems in the bone marrow microenvironment. In a dose escalation phase I clinical trial, pomalidomide showed some activity in 50% to 54% of the patients. Approximately 12% of patients developed a thrombotic event, but no other major irreversible toxicity was reported. The maximum oral tolerated dose was 4 mg/day.

Pomalidomide combined with low-dose dexamethasone has shown to be highly effective in patients with relapsed or refractory myeloma. In this study 60 patients who had previously failed two or more prior regimens, including 65% of patients relapsing after autologous transplant, received oral pomalidomide 4 mg/day on days 1 to 28, and oral dexamethasone 40 mg/day on days 1, 8, 15, and 22. All patients received aspirin 325 mg every day. With a median follow-up of 4 months, 58% of patients achieved a response with one patient having achieved a CR. Responses were seen also in 29% of 13 patients who had previously received and failed lenalidomide.

A phase III randomized multicenter study in Europe comparing the safety and efficacy of pomalidomide and low-dose dexamethasone versus solely high-dose dexamethasone showed significantly longer progression-free survival in the group receiving the pomalidomide. Additionally, several phase II trials have evaluated the use of pomalidomide in patients with myeloma that are refractory to bortezomib (see below) and/or lenalidomide. A phase III (MM-003) trial evaluated the clinical benefit of pomalidomide in combination with low-dose dexamethasone compared with high-dose dexamethasone in myeloma patients with refractory disease who had failed both bortezomib and lenalidomide therapy. In this study, the overall response rate (ORR) for patients in the pomalidomide arm was 31% versus 10% in the high-dose dexamethasone arm. Additional phase III trials evaluating pomalidomide along with low-dose dexamethasone in combination with other agents are ongoing and results are awaited. The FDA approved pomalidomide in 2013 for use in combination with dexamethasone in relapsed or refractory patients who have received at least two prior therapies including lenalidomide and bortezomib.

Pomalidomide is generally given by mouth at 4 mg per day for the first 21 days of a 4-week cycle. Most commonly observed side effects to pomalidomide include: anemia, neutropenia, thrombocytopenia, fatigue, constipation or diarrhea, peripheral neuropathy, elevated blood glucose, insomnia, and infection.

▶ Proteasome Inhibitors

Proteasome inhibitors are drugs that inhibit the function of cellular proteasomes, which are cellular protein complexes that play a role in routine protein degradation. They function to prevent the breakdown of protein in myeloma cells, leading to cell death. The ubiquitin-proteasome pathway refers to a cellular pathway that is involved in the degradation of many regulatory proteins by proteasomes. These regulatory proteins help mediate cell apoptosis, DNA repair, and cell signaling, among others. Therefore, the ubiquitin-proteasome pathway plays a vital role in maintaining the normal health of the cell. The disruption of this pathway in myeloma cells through the action of proteasome inhibition is a powerful mechanism for inducing the death of myeloma cells. The proteasome inhibitors available for the treatment of myeloma are summarized below.

Bortezomib (Velcade©)

Bortezomib is a potent proteasome inhibitor. A unique function of bortezomib is to block the nuclear factor κB (NF-κB). This factor is very important for the survival of all cells and it is also important for the development of tumor drug resistance. Normally, NF-κB is bound to its inhibitor (IkB) and NF-κB becomes free and active only when a cell receives the signal to proliferate and divide. In malignant cells, the signal for proliferating and dividing is always turned on.

Bortezomib temporarily turns off this signal such that cancer cells halt proliferation and division. Malignant cells are more sensitive to proteasome inhibition than normal cells.

Bortezomib also works by altering the production of cytokines (IL-6), growth factors (IGF-1), and angiogenesis factors (VEGF), and by inhibiting adhesion of MM cells to bone marrow stromal cells. The first clinical study to demonstrate the activity of bortezomib in multiple myeloma was conducted by Robert Orlowski and his colleagues at the MD Anderson Cancer Center in 2002. The successful results obtained in this study were confirmed in two subsequent phase II clinical studies (SUMMIT and CREST) and in a large randomized phase III trial (APEX). In May of 2003, the FDA approved bortezomib for the treatment of relapsed and refractory multiple myeloma patients who have failed two or more prior regimens.

In the APEX study, a large study involving 95 hospitals and several hundreds of patients with relapsed myeloma, patients were randomized to receive bortezomib in combination with dexamethasone versus dexamethasone alone. The response rate as well as the duration of response was higher and more durable for patients receiving the combination of drugs. Subsequent analysis showed that bortezomib could be safely administered in patients with kidney failure, including patients on hemodialysis. Bortezomib is also effective in controlling myeloma in patients with poor prognostic factors, such as elevated B2-microglobulin and unfavorable cytogenetic abnormalities.

In 2005, the FDA approved the use of bortezomib for treatment of patients with myeloma who have received at least one prior therapy. Bortezomib in combination with other anti-MM agents is currently used in patients with newly diagnosed as well as relapsed myeloma. The recommended dose of bortezomib is 1.3 mg/m^2, administered intravenously or subcutaneously twice a week for 2 weeks (days 1, 4, 8, and 11) followed by a 10-day rest period. Several studies have also explored the weekly administration schedule (days 1, 8, and 15) followed by a 10-day rest period with comparable results.

The most common side effects of bortezomib include fatigue, generalized weakness, dizziness, decreased appetite, weight loss, nausea, vomiting, diarrhea or constipation, fever, headache, cough, and occasionally hypotension. Some patients experience psychiatric disorders such as depression. Bortezomib can also cause reversible myelosuppression (suppression of bone marrow activity). Thrombocytopenia (low platelet count) occurs in the majority of patients. Concomitant antiviral prophylaxis[50] (acyclovir) is strongly recommended in patients receiving bortezomib due to an increased incidence of varicella zoster infection.[51] One-third to half of patients receiving bortezomib will experience peripheral neuropathy, with painful and abnormal sensation of hands, legs, and feet. Improvement of symptoms is often seen after dose reduction or cessation of bortezomib. Peripheral neuropathy is with certainty, the most serious side effect of bortezomib.

In 2012, the FDA approved bortezomib to be given as a subcutaneous administration (injection into fat just below the skin). The decision was based on results of a phase III study comparing subcutaneous and intravenous administration of bortezomib for myeloma patients. The results of this study showed that subcutaneous bortezomib is as effective as intravenous bortezomib, but subcutaneous administration reduces the frequency and seriousness of side effects, particularly the peripheral neuropathy.

Carfilzomib (Kyprolis©)

Carfilzomib is a selective and irreversible proteasome inhibitor with activity against bortezomib-resistant myeloma cells. Studies have indicated that carfilzomib elicits durable responses in relapsed and refractory myeloma patients. In two phase I dose escalation studies, and a single-arm phase II study, the novel agent was well tolerated with no evidence of painful peripheral neuropathy noted as well as an overall response of 35%. Responses were higher in patients who have not previously received bortezomib therapy, 57% versus 18%. A phase III trial (ENDEAVOR) of 929 patients comparing patients who received either carfilzomib or bortezomib in combination with

---

50 Concomitant antiviral prophylaxis refers to the accompanying use of antiviral medication alongside a primary drug in order to reduce risk of viral infection associated with the primary drug.

51 Varicella zoster infection is a viral infection that can cause chickenpox and shingles.

low-dose dexamethasone showed a progression-free survival of 19 months in the carfilzomib arm compared with 9 months in the bortezomib arm. Results from this study led to the FDA approval of carfilzomib.

Carfilzomib is currently approved with low-dose dexamethasone or with lenalidomide and low-dose dexamethasone for patients who have received between one and three prior treatments based on the results of the ASPIRE study. ASPIRE was a phase III study of 792 patients that compared relapsed or refractory patients receiving carfilzomib in combination with lenalidomide and dexamethasone against patients receiving a placebo in combination with lenalidomide and dexamethasone. In this study progression-free survival (PFS) was significantly longer in the group that received carfilzomib (26.3 months) versus the group that received placebo (17.6 months). With longer follow-up both studies (ENDEAVOR and ASPIRE) have displayed a survival advantage in favor of the carfilzomib arm.

Carfilzomib is administered intravenously over 30 minutes at the dose of 20 mg/m^2 on first 2 days of the first week. The dosage can be increased to 27 mg/m^2 or 56 mg/m^2 based on the dosing regimen. The most common toxicities observed are myelosuppression, fatigue, nausea, and vomiting. Less commonly, but more serious side effects such as pulmonary hypertension, heart complications, and shortness of breath have been observed. Several phase III studies are currently ongoing investigating carfilzomib in combination with other novel agents, and these results are awaited with interest.

Ixazomib (Ninlaro©)

Ixazomib is a second-generation proteasome inhibitor for use in multiple myeloma. It is administered orally, and studies have shown an increased efficacy when compared to bortezomib. Like bortezomib, it functions to induce myeloma cell death by disrupting the normal function of protein metabolism that these cells need in order to survive. Phase I/II studies have confirmed its effectiveness and safety as a single agent in relapsed or refractory patients, as well as patients who were refractory to bortezomib. Additionally, its use in combination with lenalidomide and dexamethasone as a frontline treatment has reported excellent results as well.

A phase III study (TOURMALINE-MM1) of 722 patients compared relapsed or refractory patients receiving ixazomib in combination with lenalidomide and dexamethasone against patients receiving a placebo in combination with lenalidomide and dexamethasone. In this study progression-free survival (PFS) was significantly longer in the group that received ixazomib (20.6 months) versus the group that received placebo (14.7 months). The FDA approved ixazomib in 2015 based on the positive results of this phase III study. Ixazomib is approved for use in combination with lenalidomide and dexamethasone to treat patients who have received at least one prior therapy. The results of additional phase III trials further investigating ixazomib in combination with other agents for the treatment of relapsed or refractory myeloma are awaited with interest.

The recommended dosage for ixazomib is 4 mg once a week for the first 3 weeks of every 4-week cycle. Side effects can include nausea, vomiting, diarrhea, fatigue, and rash. Unlike bortezomib, severe peripheral neuropathy due to ixazomib is rare, making it an attractive option for patients unable to tolerate bortezomib due to severe peripheral neuropathy.

▶ Histone Deacetylase Inhibitors

Histone deacetylase (HDAC) inhibitors are drugs that interfere with histone deacetylases, which are enzymes that regulate DNA expression[52] in cells. The inhibition of HDACs has been shown to result in myeloma cell death. There is evidence that HDAC inhibitors also function in part, as angiogenesis inhibitors, limiting the growth of new blood vessels to the myeloma cells. Additionally, it has been suggested that HDAC inhibitors may have effects on the immune system as well.

Panobinostat (Farydak©)

Panobinostat is the first HDAC inhibitor approved for use in multiple myeloma in combination with bortezomib and dexamethasone, for patients with relapsed or refractory myeloma who have received at

---

52 DNA expression refers to the processes by which information from a portion of DNA is used to produce a functional protein or non-protein product.

least two prior therapies consisting of bortezomib and an IMiD. Phase I/II studies have demonstrated its safety as a single agent in relapsed or refractory patients, but its activity as a single agent was found to be limited. However, preclinical support using the combination of panobinostat and bortezomib demonstrated synergy with these two agents. PANORAMA 2 was a two-stage single-arm study of the combination of panobinostat, bortezomib, and dexamethasone in patients with multiple myeloma that were refractory to bortezomib and had received at least two prior lines of treatment (median four prior regimens). This phase II trial explored whether the synergy observed with panobinostat and bortezomib could overcome chemoresistance.[53] In this study the overall response rate (ORR) was 34.5%, demonstrating increased activity of panobinostat when used in combination with bortezomib. A phase III study (PANORAMA 1) of 768 heavily pretreated patients showed that patients treated with the combination of panobinostat, dexamethasone, and bortezomib significantly extended progression-free survival (12 months) when compared to patients treated with dexamethasone and bortezomib alone (8.1 months).

The FDA approved panobinostat in 2015, in combination with bortezomib and dexamethasone, for patients who have received at least two prior standard therapies. Unfortunately, the toxicity observed with this regimen can be significant. Panobinostat is administered orally, and the recommended dose is 20 mg taken orally once every other day for three doses per week, on weeks 1 and 2 of each 21-day cycle. Side effects of panobinostat include: peripheral edema, fever, diarrhea, nausea, vomiting, and fatigue. Less commonly, cardiac toxicity, severely low platelet count, severely low red blood cell count, liver problems, severe diarrhea, and infection have been observed.

▶ Monoclonal Antibodies

Monocolonal antibodies are a newer class of drugs that are being investigated for use in the treatment of myeloma. They are produced in the lab and mimic the antibodies our own immune systems

---

53 Chemoresistance refers to the resistance of malignant cells to certain antimyeloma medications or treatments.

produce in response to foreign substances that enter our bodies. Each group of monoclonal antibodies is made up of identical duplicate copies of a specific type of antibody, hence the term monoclonal, or one type. The monoclonal antibodies studied for use in multiple myeloma treatment both recognize and attach to specific proteins expressed on myeloma cells. Each group of monoclonal antibodies is designed for their own specific protein expressed by the myeloma cell. Currently, they have been studied primarily in patients with relapsed and refractory disease. Monoclonal antibodies have been shown to be active against myeloma even in patients with highly unfavorable cytogenetic abnormalities that are either initially present, or acquired over time. The success of this class of drugs represents an important shift in the way we are able treat multiple myeloma.

Elotuzumab (Empliciti©)

Elotuzumab is a first-generation immune therapy monoclonal antibody for use in patients with multiple myeloma. This monoclonal antibody targets an antigen molecule known as SLAMF7,[54] which is expressed on both myeloma and NK (natural killer) cells. Elotuzumab works against myeloma cells in two major ways. First, elotuzumab serves to further activate NK cell activity by interacting with SLAMF7 expressed on NK cells. Second, this monoclonal antibody interacts with SLAMF7 expressed on myeloma cells to activate antibody-dependent cellular cytotoxicity (ADCC),[55] resulting in myeloma cell destruction. Thus, elotuzumab works to both directly target myeloma cells, as well as enhance NK cell activity against myeloma cells.

A phase II trial with elotuzumab in combination with lenalidomide and low-dose dexamethasone showed encouraging results in patients with relapsed disease, as well as in patients with unfavorable cytogenetics. A phase III randomized study (ELOQUENT-2) of 646 patients with relapsed or refractory myeloma showed that the combination of

---

54 SLAMF7 is a protein targeted by elotuzumab that is expressed on the surface of nearly all myeloma cells as well as some types of immune cells.

55 Antibody-dependent cellular cytotoxicity (ADCC) refers to the destruction of an antibody-coated target cell by short-lived cells of the immune system called effector cells.

lenalidomide, dexamethasone, and elotuzumab resulted in a significant improvement in overall response rate as well as an increase in progression-free survival (PFS) (19.4 vs. 14.8 months) when compared to patients receiving lenalidomide and dexamethasone alone.

The FDA approved eolotuzumab in 2015 for relapsed or refractory patients in combination with lenalidomide and dexamethasone. Elotuzumab appears to work synergistically with lenalidomide and pomalidomide in order to provide a more efficacious response. It is given intravenously, and though the optimal dosage is still being studied, patients have been treated with 10 mg/kg as well as 20 mg/kg. The recommended dose is 10 mg/kg intravenously every week for the first two cycles and every 2 weeks thereafter. Common side effects of elotuzumab are primarily infusion related and include: nausea, headache, fatigue, fever, and dizziness. Less commonly observed side effects can include low red and white blood cell counts, diarrhea, and low potassium levels. Further studies investigating the use of elotuzumab in other combinations of treatment will provide further insight into the utility of this drug.

Daratumumab (Darzlex©)

Daratumumab is another first-generation immune therapy monoclonal antibody for use in patients with multiple myeloma. This monoclonal antibody targets CD38, an antigen molecule that is highly expressed on myeloma cells. CD38 is a cell surface protein that is involved in cellular messenger pathways that regulate myeloma cell survival, death, and proliferation. Daratumumab mediates both complement-dependent cytotoxicity (CDC)[56] and antibody-dependent cellular cytotoxicity (ADCC) against myeloma cells.

Most studies to date have investigated daratumumab as a single agent. A phase II study in patients in refractory myeloma patients showed an increased 1-year overall survival rate and overall response rate after administration of daratumumab as a monotherapy (single agent). When studied in combination with lenalidomide and dexamethasone, the overall response rate was significantly higher.

---

56 Complement-dependent cytotoxicity (CDC) refers to a process that recruits specialized immune cell proteins (complement proteins) to destroy a target cell.

A combined analysis of 148 patients who had received a median of five prior therapies, treated with daratumumab alone at 16 mg/kg, reported an impressive overall response rate of 31%.

The FDA granted accelerated approval for daratumumab in 2015 for patients who have received at least three prior treatments. A phase III study (CASTOR) comparing patients receiving daratumumab, bortezomib, and dexamethasone versus bortezomib and dexamethasone in patients with relapsed or refractory multiple myeloma showed an increase in overall response rate (ORR) as well as PFS for the daratumumab arm. Similarly another phase III study (POLLUX) comparing patients receiving daratumumab, lenalidomide, and dexamethasone versus lenalidomide and dexamethasone in patients with relapsed or refractory myeloma showed a significant increase in progression-free survival and a higher percentage of minimal residual disease (MRD) negative patients in the daratumumab arm.

In 2017 the FDA approved daratumumab in combination with lenalidomide and/or bortezomib in first relapse, as well as daratumumab in combination with pomalidomide for patients who have failed at least two lines of treatment. Daratumumab is given intravenously, and the recommended dosage is 16 mg per kilogram of body weight. Infusions are given once a week for the first 8 weeks of treatment, once every 2 weeks from weeks 9 to 24, and once every 4 weeks from week 24 onwards. Like elotuzumab, side effects are primarily infusion related and can include: fever, fatigue, nausea, blood pressure changes, thrombocytopenia, anemia, low white blood cell levels, and elevated liver enzymes. Further studies of daratumumab in combination with various other therapies as well as administration in a subcutaneous formulation are awaited with interest.

▶ Treatment Overview

The following section will provide a highly generalized overview of the treatment for patients with multiple myeloma. Due to the rate at which therapies are being introduced into the clinic as well as the rate at which currently accepted guidelines are being amended, we will refrain from going into specifics regarding the current drug combinations used in the newly diagnosed and relapsed settings. Current information can be found at www.myeloma.org/understanding /10-steps/treatment and www.themmrf.org.

As new drugs are approved and the treatment landscape evolves, new combinations of treatments are being approved for the newly diagnosed as well as the relapsed disease setting. Many factors are to be taken in consideration prior to initiating treatment for patients with multiple myeloma such as the age of the patient, the presence of specific symptoms, the overall general health, and the performance status. For example, patients with severe pain due to bone involvement might require treatment with localized radiotherapy before starting systemic therapy. Preserving the patient's lifestyle and maintaining a good quality of life should be priorities. The more recently introduced agents, such as thalidomide, lenalidomide, and bortezomib, have gained favor over the more traditional and more toxic chemotherapy drugs. Stem cell transplant[57] (see Chapter 5) remains the initial choice for the majority of patients in good performance status and if the newer agents will eventually replace transplant remains the primary focus of many current debates.

The development of the previously described novel targeted agents over the last decade have led to innovative and effective treatment options to all patients with myeloma, both those proceeding to transplant and those not deemed transplant candidates. Studies to determine the most effective and least toxic combinations as well as their optimal schedules and doses are currently underway. Choosing the best treatment for each individual patient requires careful discussions between patients, their families, and physicians as well as a continuous and careful review of all the emerging new information and data.

The term relapse is used to describe the reappearance of myeloma protein and/or myeloma symptoms in patients who were previously in complete remission. The term progression is used to describe an increase of myeloma protein and/or myeloma symptoms in patients who were previously in partial remission. The term refractory is used to describe patients not responding to therapy or progressing within 60 days of their last therapy. For many years the standard treatment for multiple myeloma was an oral alkylator agent, melphalan given in combination with a steroid pill, prednisone (M&P). The two drugs were administered for approximately 1 week at the beginning of each

---

57 Stem cell transplant refers to a procedure that infuses healthy blood stem cells from an individual's own body or from a donor, into the individual's body to replace damaged or diseased bone marrow.

month. Therapy was continued for many months sometimes up to a year, or until the patient had evidence of disease progression. At time of relapse or at time of progression, patients were treated with a more aggressive combination of chemotherapeutic drugs administered mostly in the vein.

The first report that high doses of melphalan given intravenously could work for patients with relapsed myeloma was published in 1983. In this study 11 patients with advanced myeloma were treated with high-dose melphalan and they all responded. Later, Dr. Bart Barlogie introduced the use of stem cell transplant to rescue patients after high-dose chemotherapy. High-dose melphalan and stem cell transplant remains today an acceptable and valid treatment option not only for patients with newly diagnosed myeloma but also for patients with relapsed or refractory myeloma. However, the recent introduction of several novel agents such as lenalidomide, bortezomib, carfilzomib, ixazomib, daratumumab, pomalidomide, panobinostat, and elotuzumab, among others, has changed the treatment paradigm for patients with relapsed or refractory disease. Over the last few years a large number of innovative regimens have been proposed, and numerous regimens are currently under investigation in clinical trials. Patients who don't respond to a specific agent can respond to the same agent given at a different dose, or when given in combination with drugs that have other mechanisms of action.

In summary, over the last several years many new drugs have been tested and subsequently approved for the treatment of multiple myeloma. Understanding the biology of this disease has helped researchers to identify new drugs, clarify their mechanisms of action, better define their potential side effects, and devise new and more potent combinations of drugs to treat MM. New drugs will increasingly be approved for multiple myeloma as the treatment landscape for MM continues to evolve rapidly. For more information regarding currently approved drugs, dosing, and clinical evidence, please visit www.themmrf.org /multiple-myeloma-knowledge-center/myeloma-drugs-guide/.

In the remaining chapters, we will focus on the specifics of high-dose chemotherapy and stem cell transplantation, distinguishing transplant and non-transplant candidates, supportive care therapies, and emerging therapies.

CHAPTER 5

High-Dose Chemotherapy and Stem Cell Transplant

▶ Introduction to Blood and Marrow Transplants

For many populations of myeloma patients, particularly those who are younger or in good performance status,[1] the most aggressive approaches to treatment should be considered. The most aggressive approaches typically involve giving the patient high-dose therapies (HDT), which may be more effective than lower doses of chemotherapy due to the more pronounced effects. High-dose therapies can include administration of high doses of chemotherapy drugs like melphalan and sometimes, high doses of radiation to the entire body. Unfortunately, while high-dose chemotherapy attacks myeloma cells, it can also destroy normal blood-producing cells called hematopoietic stem cells. Therefore, patients who receive HDT also need to receive a transplant of healthy blood stem cells after the HDT is given in order to restore the production of healthy blood cells. When the stem cells come from a patient's own bone marrow, it is called an autologous transplant. When the stem cells come from another person, it is called an allogeneic transplant. In the next sections, the procedures, risks, and potential benefits of high-dose therapy followed by either an autologous or allogeneic stem cell transplant will be discussed.

---

1 Performance status describes a patient's level of functionality with respect to his or her physical ability, daily activity, and ability to care for him- or herself.

▶ Steps in an Autologous Stem Cell Transplant

Collection of Hematopoietic Stem Cells

Most stem cells are found in the bone marrow, but they can also be found in the peripheral blood as well as in the blood within a newborn's umbilical cord.[2] Up until the mid-1990s, almost all transplants used stem cells taken directly from the bone marrow, termed a bone marrow harvest. When the stem cells are taken directly from the bone marrow, the liquid portion of the marrow is collected using a needle inserted in the bone. This procedure is called a bone marrow aspiration. In order to collect enough stem cells, the donor needs to undergo many bone marrow aspirations over about an hour to an hour and a half, under general anesthesia in the operating room. The stem cells can then be frozen (cryopreserved), and they can be stored for many years, if necessary. Side effects of this procedure include local pain that lasts 1 to 2 weeks for most persons and more rarely, bleeding, nerve damage, and infections.

Currently, the majority of transplants use stem cells collected from the blood. Under normal conditions, only very low numbers of stem cells are circulating in the blood. Therefore, in order to collect a sufficient number of stem cells from the peripheral blood, it is necessary to move them from the bone marrow into the bloodstream. This procedure is called stem cell mobilization,[3] and requires that patients receive a medication that increases the number of stem cells in the bloodstream. The most common medication currently used to mobilize stem cells is called a granulocyte-colony stimulating factor (G-CSF, or Neupogen).[4] G-CSF is usually injected under the skin for 4-5 days prior to the stem cell collection.

---

2 Umbilical cord is a cord that carries oxygen and nutrients from the mother's placenta into the baby's bloodstream. The blood within is rich in stem cells that can be collected after childbirth.

3 Stem cell mobilization refers to the recruitment of hematopoietic stem cells from the bone marrow into the peripheral blood for collection.

4 Granulocyte-colony stimulating factor (G-CSF) is a protein that stimulates the bone marrow to produce and release stem cells into the bloodstream.

For patients who failed to mobilize using G-CSF alone, Mozobil© (plerixafor injection) is approved by the US Food and Drug Administration (FDA) to be used with G-CSF to mobilize hematopoietic stem cell into the peripheral blood for collection in patients with non-Hodgkin's lymphoma (NHL) or multiple myeloma (MM). Mozobil©, in combination with G-CSF, releases hematopoietic stem cells from the bone marrow into the blood by disrupting a connection between stem cells and the bone marrow stroma. The most common adverse reactions observed during stem cells mobilization with Mozobil© are: diarrhea (37%), nausea (34%), tiredness (fatigue) (27%), injection site reactions (34%), headache (22%), pain in the joints (arthralgia) (13%), dizziness (11%), and vomiting (10%).

A chemotherapy drug such as cyclophosphamide can be given prior to G-CSF in order to help mobilize stem cells. This strategy is called cyclophosphamide priming. While cyclophosphamide priming initially has myelosuppressive effects, this is followed by a stimulation of the bone marrow to produce more stem cells. Cyclophosphamide priming allows for a more effective collection, as well as the collection of potentially increased amounts of stem cells, when compared to G-CSF treatment alone. This medication may also help further treat the myeloma before transplant, but the side effects of such an approach have to be carefully considered. Once the stem cells have been mobilized from the bone marrow into the blood, they are collected through a procedure called leukapheresis[5] (or pheresis). Intravenous (IV) lines are placed either in the arms (if the veins are big enough) or into a large vein in the neck or under the collarbone. Blood is then circulated through the IV lines through a machine called an apheresis device. With this machine the stem cells can be separated from the other blood cells and collected in a bag. The rest of the blood is given back to the patient through the IV lines. The pheresis procedure usually last several hours, during which time donors typically are able to watch television or read a book. Once the stem cells are collected, they are cryopreserved for use later in the autologous transplant.

---

5 Leukapheresis is a laboratory procedure in which a particular component of blood is separated out, and the rest of the blood is reintroduced back into the circulation.

Enough stem cells may be collected in one session or it may require repeating the pheresis procedure several days in a row. Most patients yield sufficient stem cells for an autologous transplant but prior chemotherapy, particularly melphalan or prolonged exposure with lenalidomide, may lessen the yield. If not enough stem cells are collected using pheresis, some patients may be asked to consider a bone marrow harvest as an alternative. Side effects of pheresis include bone or back pain caused by the G-CSF (due to increased blood cell production from the bone marrow), lip tingling, and other symptoms due to low blood calcium levels during the pheresis procedure (caused by the anticoagulant[6] used when the stem cells are collected) and rarely, bleeding, infections, and lung and nerve damage from placement of the IV lines.

High-Dose Therapy Administration

Once enough hematopoietic stem cells are collected and frozen, the patient rests for 1 to 2 weeks before proceeding to treatment with high-dose chemotherapy. When high-dose chemotherapy is administered prior to a stem cell transplant, it is also called the preparative or conditioning regimen.[7] The rationale for using high-dose therapy is that for most people, it destroys a large number of myeloma cells with a single treatment. High-dose melphalan given alone or in combination with total body irradiation (TBI)[8] were the most commonly used conditioning regimens for patients with myeloma in the 1990s. Because patients treated with TBI experience more side effects than patients treated with high-dose melphalan alone, and their response rate is similar, based on the results of a large randomized study comparing melphalan alone vs. melphalan/TBI, most transplant physicians prefer to use only melphalan. The effect of melphalan appears to be dose dependent. The recommended dose of melphalan used as conditioning regimen is 200 mg/m^2 given in a vein over a period of 30 minutes.

---

6 Anticoagulant is a substance that helps to prevent the clotting of blood.

7 Preparative or conditioning regimen refers to a therapy or combination of therapies used to prepare an individual for transplant.

8 Total body irradiation (TBI) is a form of radiation therapy that incorporates the entire body, generally in preparation for a stem cell transplant.

The dose of melphalan is generally adjusted for patients with renal disease and patients older than 70. Other chemotherapy agents such as busulfan, cyclophosphamide, and carmustine (see Chapter 4) have been used as conditioning regimens but it is still unclear if any of those drugs may improve the effects observed with melphalan alone.

Stem Cell Reinfusion and Engraftment

One or two days after high-dose chemotherapy, patients will receive the stem cells back using an IV inserted in the neck or chest. After they are reinfused, the stem cells will travel through the blood into the bone marrow and will start to restore the marrow and produce new blood cells in approximately 2 weeks. This process is called engraftment.[9] During this time, patients will likely receive antibiotics to fight infections, as their immune system is still in a compromised state. If necessary, they may also receive blood cell or platelet transfusions until the transplanted stem cells start to produce new blood cells. In many treatment centers patients may receive their high-dose chemotherapy, stem cell reinfusion, and care following the transplant, on an outpatient[10] basis rather than in a hospital setting. However, patients need to stay very close to the treatment center so they can be seen and monitored as frequently as every day until they are fully recovered.

Many centers also require that patients receiving outpatient treatment have a caregiver, who is a close family member or friend who can assist in transportation, minor medical care, and can phone the doctor or nurse on call if any problems develop. Less than one-third of patients who start their treatment as an outpatient require admission to the hospital for a brief period of time if a serious infection or other problem develops. The majority of patients are able to complete the entire treatment as an outpatient. Some who have other medical problems in addition to myeloma, or don't have a caregiver, may require admission to the hospital for the entire treatment even if the center offers outpatient treatment to patients.

---

9 Engraftment is the process by which transplanted stem cells migrate to the patient's bone marrow from the peripheral blood in order to begin producing blood cells.

10 Outpatient refers to patients who receive medical treatment in a clinic without being admitted to a hospital.

▶ Risks and Potential Side Effects of Autologous Transplant

The most common complications or side effects occur within 5 to 10 days from the day the high-dose melphalan is given. These include complete suppression of the production of the blood cells, mouth sores (called oral mucositis), nausea, vomiting, diarrhea, hair loss, skin rash, infections, and bleeding. These side effects result from the drug's particularly potent activity against all fast-growing cells in the body, which can encompass cells of the entire gastrointestinal tract from the mouth to anus, hair follicles, and blood-producing cells. The majority of patients will experience moderate to severe mouth sores and mouth pain, and some patients will not be able to eat solid food for a least a week or so after transplant. Other complications that occur much less frequently include kidney, lung, liver, and/or heart problems. Many of these problems get better once the new blood cells start to be made, somewhere between 10–21 days after the reinfusion of the stem cells. Occasionally some side effects, including infections and organ damage, can take weeks to months to resolve. Very rarely, some patients experience lifelong organ damage from the treatment. Depression, cataracts, infertility, and other cancers may occur months to years later. The risk of dying in the first days and weeks after an autologous stem cell transplant is approximately 1%–2%, though this percentage can vary among treatment centers with more or less experience performing the procedure. Death can be a result of a life-threatening infection, major bleeding, strokes or blood clots, damage to the heart, liver or kidneys, or other complications of the high-dose chemotherapy. We reiterate that the risk of death is lower if the stem cell transplant is performed in a medical center that has significant experience with performing this procedure.

Who Is a Good Autologous Transplant Candidate?

Many factors must be taken in consideration to determine whether a patient is a good transplant candidate. A transplant candidate is generally a younger patient who is in adequate general health and suitable level of fitness. Older patients in good general health and good performance status can also proceed to transplant if the doctor determines that high-dose therapy could be beneficial and relatively safe for them. A doctor who specializes in stem cell transplant should evaluate and ultimately decide if a patient is a good transplant candidate. The decision that the transplant is the best course of action should be made jointly between the doctor and the patient, along with his/her family.

What Are the Potential Benefits of Autologous Transplantation?

Higher dose therapy (HDT) followed by autologous stem cell transplant improves the rates of complete remission (depth of response) and can prolong the duration of remission and the life of patients with myeloma. High-dose therapy and stem cell transplant has been used to treat multiple myeloma for more than 30 years. In fact, the first evidence that high-dose melphalan could be used to rescue patients with relapsed myeloma was published in 1983. In this small study, 11 patients with relapsed or refractory myeloma who had already received many prior regimens were treated with high-dose melphalan and they all showed some evidence of response. Because high-dose intravenous melphalan causes profound suppression of blood cell manufacture, Dr. Bart Barlogie and his colleagues introduced stem cell transplant as a rescue technique. However, these initial studies were either small, or larger but not randomized.[11] The French group, Intergroup Francais du Myeloma (IFM), was the first to conduct a randomized clinical trial that showed that high-dose therapy followed by autologous transplant was superior to conventional chemotherapy. In this study reported in 1996, 200 patients with newly diagnosed MM were randomized to receive either a short course of induction therapy followed by high-dose therapy and stem cell transplant, or conventional chemotherapy only. This study clearly showed that the patients in the high-dose therapy group not only lived longer but also had a prolonged period free of myeloma.

---

11 Randomized studies are clinical trials in which the individuals being studied are assigned, by chance, to separate groups that compare different treatments. Neither the researchers nor the participants serve to influence to which group the individuals are assigned.

These findings were confirmed by a second large randomized study of 407 patients conducted in the United Kingdom. Subsequently, other large studies of high-dose therapy and autologous stem cell transplant were published in the literature; some were randomized and others were not. Not all those studies showed that high-dose therapy is better than conventional therapy for prolonging the life of myeloma patients. However, the majority of those studies showed that patients who achieved a complete remission after high-dose therapy and transplant lived longer free of myeloma, and hence without the need of additional chemotherapy or other treatment until the time of relapse. The majority of patients who respond to high-dose therapy and stem cell transplant remain in remission for few years. A number of patients may remain in remission for a longer period of time, and a few have lived in remission for up to 10 years after transplant. High-dose therapy followed by stem cell transplant allows some patients to remain not only myeloma free but also free from further aggressive treatment for a few years and sometimes longer.

In addition to using autologous transplant as part of the initial treatment of myeloma, it can also be offered later to patients with myeloma when they relapse from some other form of initial treatment. A large randomized study of 202 patients conducted in France was designed to answer the question: is transplant better earlier or later in the course of the disease? This study showed that the chance of responding to high-dose therapy was very similar for both groups of patients. However, it also showed that the quality of life of patients receiving transplant sooner after diagnosis was better. This is mainly due to the fact that the patients who were transplanted later overall had received more chemotherapy, which affected their quality of life. Additionally, this study showed that the period without myeloma was longer if transplant was done sooner.

While the majority of the randomized studies of high-dose therapy and autologous stem cell transplant reported in the literature were designed for patients under the age of 65, several nonrandomized[12]

---

12 Nonrandomized trials are studies in which the individuals being studied are either assigned to a particular treatment group or are able to choose to which treatment group they wish to be assigned.

studies were reported and confirmed that high-dose therapy and autologous transplant is also well tolerated in patients older than age 65. As a result, many treatment centers do not have an upper age limit for performing autologous transplantation in MM, but try to weigh the risks and benefits of this aggressive treatment for each individual patient.

The role of high-dose therapy (HDT) followed by autologous stem cell transplantation (ASCT) has recently been questioned due to unprecedented success that has been achieved with the newer treatments. Major studies comparing newer agents to high-dose therapy and stem cell transplant are ongoing, though data from four large studies have been reported in the literature. While so far all four randomized published clinical studies have supported the benefit in terms of duration of remission for HDT followed by ASCT early on, a few of these studies have suggested no benefit to the patient's overall survival. This being said, the follow-up of these patients is still too short to make a final determination.

The most important of these studies, lead by Dr. Michel Attal, was published in the *New England Journal of Medicine* in April 2017. In this study 700 patients with newly diagnosed multiple myeloma were randomized to receive a short course of induction therapy with three cycles of RVD (lenalidomide/bortezomib/dexamethasone) and then additional therapy with either five more cycles of RVD or high-dose melphalan plus ASCT followed by two additional cycles of RVD. Of note, ~70% of patients who didn't receive transplant early on underwent transplant later at time of disease relapse, a factor that makes the impact of ASCT on overall survival almost impossible to assess. Patients in both groups received maintenance therapy with lenalidomide for 1 year. The primary end point was progression-free survival (duration of response). Median progression-free survival was significantly longer in the group that underwent transplantation early than in the group that received RVD alone (50 months vs. 36 months). In addition, the number of patients achieving a complete response was higher in the early transplantation group than in the RVD-alone group as was the number of patients with minimal residual disease negative (MRD-neg). Overall survival at 4 years did not differ significantly between the transplantation group and the RVD-alone group (81% and 82%, respectively); however once again we must remember that 70% of the patients in the *nontransplant* group received transplant later on and that longer follow-up is needed.

This study was initiated several years ago as collaboration between the IMF (French Myeloma Intergroup led by Dr. Attal) and the US. Those patients treated in the US were entered into the *DETERMINATION Study* led by Dr. Paul Richardson at the Dana-Farber Cancer Institute. The main difference in the patients treated on this study in France versus the US was the duration of maintenance therapy with lenalidomide, 1 year (France) versus until disease progression or toxicity (US). Whether longer continuation of therapy with lenalidomide will make a difference in the results of the study remains to be seen. It is important to note that all these studies are examining the best timing of transplant "early vs. delay," as transplant still remains a key intervention even in this era of the new-targeted therapies in the fight against myeloma.

Until the information from these studies is clear based on long-term follow-up, many treatment centers continue to recommend that for most patients, initial treatment of myeloma includes induction therapy for a short period of time followed by high-dose therapy and autologous stem cell transplantation. For now, even in our current era of novel treatments, transplant appears to remain beneficial and should be considered as standard of care for all patients in good performance status.

For those patients who are not transplant candidates because of age or other medical problems, other treatments may be recommended instead. Lastly, because no treatment can be depended on to definitively cure myeloma and it remains unclear what the best treatment should be, many centers offer a variety of clinical trials designed to help determine optimal treatment of strategies.

▶ How to Improve Autologous Stem Cell Transplant Outcomes

One of the major concerns of high-dose therapy and autologous stem cell transplant is that eventually, nearly all myeloma patients will relapse. Therefore, many new and innovative strategies have been evaluated in order to improve the outcome of stem cell transplant, and some of these strategies are currently under investigation. Several of these strategies are summarized below.

"Purging" the Autologous Stem Cells

One of the many reasons patients relapse after high-dose therapy and autologous stem cell transplant could be because their stem cells are contaminated with myeloma cells. Myeloma typically grows in the bone marrow and myeloma cells can be frequently found in the autologous bone marrow or blood stem cell collections that are frozen for the transplant. Consequently, it is possible that these contaminating myeloma cells could be reinfused back into the patient at the time the healthy stem cells are reinfused. This concern prompted researchers to investigate different ways to clean the stem cells in the laboratory after they are collected and prior to re-infusing them back to the patient. So far, none of the studies published in the literature showed a survival advantage for patients who had their stem cells purged.[13] In addition, during the purging process some of the beneficial stem cells are lost, which could explain why the patients who receive purged stem cells took longer to engraft and experienced a higher number of infection complications. Recently, newer purging techniques to separate the stem cells have been developed. Determining if the newer techniques are more effective will require a new generation of purging studies.

Tandem (Double) Autologous Stem Cell Transplants

The Intergroup Francais du Myelome was the first group to compare single versus tandem autologous stem cell transplant. In this study (IFM 94 trial), 399 patients younger than age 60 and with newly diagnosed myeloma were randomized to receive one versus two rounds of high-dose therapy followed by autologous stem cell transplant. After 7 years, the probability of (a) being alive (overall survival) and (b) being alive without evidence of disease (progression-free survival), were twice as high in the tandem transplant group. Further analysis showed that

---

13 Purging refers to an attempt to eradicate residual tumor cell contamination from the population of stem cells collected for transplantation.

the patients who most benefited from the second transplant were the patients that hadn't achieved a very good response after the first transplant. On the other hand, patients who had achieved a very good response after one transplant did not seem to benefit from the second transplant. Several other large studies comparing single versus double autologous transplant were subsequently initiated. So far only a couple showed results similar to the French study, and therefore, tandem autologous transplants are still not recommended for all patients with myeloma. However, it is very reasonable to collect enough stem cells for two or more autologous transplants for all patients with myeloma. Stem cells can be frozen and stored for many years. A second transplant (sometimes called a salvage transplant[14]) can be performed at the time of relapse for patients who remain in remission for longer than 24 to 36 months.

Maintenance Therapy Following Stem Cell Transplant

One strategy to keep patients from relapsing after transplant is to administer further treatment in the form of maintenance therapy.[15] In the past, studies were conducted involving the use of interferon and steroids as maintenance therapy post-transplant. These strategies are not commonly used to date due to their poor tolerability and significant toxicities in the maintenance setting. With the introduction of newer drugs including immunomodulators and proteasome inhibitors, several clinical studies were designed to investigate their role after transplant.

In the summer of 2006, the French group reported their experience of using thalidomide after tandem autologous transplant. 597 patients with newly diagnosed myeloma (age <65) received 4 months of induction therapy followed by tandem autologous stem cell transplant. Approximately 4 months after the second transplant, all the patients who had achieved a response were randomly assigned to one of three treatment groups. Patients assigned to group A were

---

14 Salvage transplant is a transplant often given to a patient whose disease relapses early, and can be used to bridge a patient to a subsequent therapy.
15 Maintenance therapy is a low-dose therapy given to patients in remission to prolong disease progression and relapse.

followed without treatment. Patients assigned to group B received monthly pamidronate,[16] and patients assigned to group C received both pamidronate and thalidomide. In this study, patients assigned to group C (pamidronate+thalidomide) lived longer than patients assigned to group A or group B. The major downside of this study was that a large number of patients in the thalidomide group had to discontinue it because adverse effects. The most notable side effects were peripheral neuropathy, fatigue, and constipation.

This study as well as others showed an improved progression-free survival (PFS) for patients on maintenance therapy with thalidomide, however it is not widely used as a maintenance therapy due to its significant cumulative toxicity.

Currently the standard of treatment for patients post-autologous transplant is to receive maintenance therapy with low-dose lenalidomide (Revlimid©). A study in 2014 assigned 251 patients to either lenalidomide maintenance therapy or no maintenance therapy post-autologous stem cell transplantation. In this study, progression-free survival was significantly prolonged (43 months vs. 22.4 months) in the group that received lenalidomide maintenance. This study and others have now confirmed its efficacy, tolerability, and relative safety as a maintenance therapy. Lenalidomide maintenance therapy prolongs duration of remission and overall survival of patients with myeloma. Based on these positive results the FDA in 2017 officially approved low-dose lenalidomide in this setting. It should be noted that long-term maintenance therapy with lenalidomide was found to result in an increased risk of developing a secondary cancer.

Finally, the use of bortezomib (Velcade©) has been investigated as an efficacious maintenance strategy in certain populations of patients with increased risk factors such as renal insufficiency, an inability to tolerate lenalidomide, and certain high-risk cytogenetic abnormalities. Two large randomized studies investigating bortezomib in the maintenance setting, published by the HOVON/GMMG group and Spanish group, showed a PFS benefit as well as relatively tolerable side effects. Unfortunately, neither of these studies compared bortezomib maintenance post-transplant to no maintenance. While

---

16 Pamidronate, or pamidronic acid, is a drug used to prevent osteoporosis (see Chapter 6).

the use of proteasome inhibitors such as bortezomib and ixazomib are still being evaluated in the maintenance setting, these and other studies have shown that it can be an effective maintenance strategy in certain populations of myeloma patients.

Ultimately, when offering maintenance therapy after autologous transplant, physicians must take into consideration any potential quality of life issues resulting from side effects of the therapy. For this reason, some physicians opt to initiate therapy after transplant only at the first sign of disease progression. Newer studies involving the use of more recently released agents such as next-generation proteasome inhibitors, immunomodulators, and immunotherapy post-transplant, as well as tailored maintenance strategies based on genetic analysis, are currently ongoing.

Combined High-Dose and Standard-Dose Chemotherapy

Efforts to innovate upon the standard chemotherapy transplant conditioning regimen of melphalan 200 mg/m^2 have not resulted in improved outcomes with acceptable toxicity to date. The most widely used conditioning regimen in preparation for autologous stem cell transplant for multiple myeloma, as described above, is a single dose of the chemotherapy drug melphalan. Several studies have investigated ways to optimize the conditioning regimen through dose intensification or the addition of total body irradiation (TBI). While reported response rates and improvements in progression-free survival have appeared promising in some studies, the toxicities and transplant-related morality (TRM) associated with these more intensive regimens have prevented their widespread adoption.

The myeloma treatment group at the University of Arkansas has pioneered a very intensive and aggressive treatment approach to myeloma, which involves receiving scheduled combinations of chemotherapy and one or more high-dose therapies with autologous transplant. This aggressive approach has been termed *total therapy,* and has gone through several generations of modifications in hopes of making it more effective and less toxic. The group in Arkansas treats many patients from around the world, but whether this approach is more effective than other less-intensive treatment approaches remains unclear.

▶ Allogeneic Stem Cell Transplants

An allogeneic transplant is a transplant of hematopoietic stem cells from a healthy donor, who may be a relative or a complete stranger who has volunteered to donate hematopoietic stem cells. Most importantly, the donor's stem cells need to genetically match the recipient's stem cells. This genetic matching is called HLA matching,[17] because it involves checking a group of genes called the HLA genes.[18] The HLA genes are critical to whether the recipient will accept or reject the transplant and whether they will develop another problem called graft-versus-host disease, which is discussed further below. HLA matching or *tissue matching* is different from blood typing, such that two people could have the same blood type but not be HLA matched, or could have different blood types and yet be HLA matched. People do not have to have the same blood type for the allogeneic transplant to work, as long as their HLA genes are matched. When the stem cells come from an identical twin, it is called syngeneic transplant. When the stem cells come from a genetically matched brother or sister, it is called an HLA-matched sibling transplant. When the stem cells come from a genetically matched volunteer donor, it is called a matched unrelated-donor (MUD) transplant.

The main advantages of an allogeneic transplant are that the donor stem cells are not contaminated with myeloma cells, and that the new immune system the patient will receive through their donor stem cell infusion may be more effective at fighting the residual disease. The proportion of patients with myeloma that achieve a complete remission after an allogeneic transplant is very high, and it appears that some of these patients may even be cured of their disease. Despite these encouraging results, high-dose therapy followed by donor stem cells re-infusion has not been widely used to treat myeloma patients because a high proportion of patients die during or immediately after transplant. The chance of dying immediately

17 HLA matching is blood testing used to match a blood or bone marrow donor to a recipient for transplant or infusion.
18 HLA genes are a group of genes that encode cell-surface proteins responsible for the regulation of the immune system.

after allogeneic transplant period has been reported to be as high as 30%–50%. The risk of death is primarily due to complications of the high-dose therapy (also known as myeloblative regimen[19]), which is much more intensive than that of an autologous transplant conditioning regimen, and to the graft-versus-host disease (GVHD).

Graft-versus-host disease (GVHD) is a common side effect of an allogeneic bone marrow or a cord blood transplant.[20] In GVHD, the immune cells from the donor attack the body of the patient. GVHD can affect many different parts of the body, with the skin, liver, and intestines most often affected. GVHD can range from mild to life threatening. Over the last several years with the introduction of new diagnostic tests and stronger supportive care, the number of patients dying during or soon after an allogeneic transplant appears to be decreasing. This observation prompted transplant physicians to revisit this option for younger myeloma patients who have a suitable donor. However, it is still preferable to treat patients with an allogeneic transplant as part of a clinical trial. Due to the high risk of dying in the immediate post-transplant period, allogeneic patients need to remain in the hospital for the first 4 to 6 weeks of transplant. After that, they need to stay close to the treatment center for an additional 2 months until they are fully recovered. Since patients receive a completely new hematopoietic system during an allogeneic transplant, donor stem cell engraftment as well as possible graft rejection[21] by the body must be carefully monitored and accounted for.

Nonmyeloablative Allogeneic Transplant

To avoid the toxicity of the high-dose chemotherapy used for an allogeneic transplant (full myeloablative transplant), in the late 1990s and the beginning of 2000, physicians started to use lower

---

19 Myeloblative regimen refers to high-dose therapy used in an allogeneic stem cell transplant to kill cancer cells in the bone marrow.
20 Cord blood transplant is a stem cell transplant in which the source of stem cells originates from umbilical cord blood that is donated by a mother after the birth of an infant.
21 Graft rejection is a situation involving a transplant recipient's own immune system attacking the transplanted tissue or organ.

dose chemotherapy to prepare patients for this type of transplant (nonmyeloablative or "mini" allogeneic transplant). The rationale behind this decision was to try to reduce the risks associated with allogeneic transplant without eliminating the benefits of having a new immune system to fight the disease. Nonmyeloablative transplants are associated with lower mortality rates and with lower toxicity or side effects. The results of some initial but relatively small studies for multiple myeloma were quite encouraging. Those studies showed that a very high proportion of patients treated with mini-allogeneic transplants could achieve a complete remission. However, this was true only for patients who had stable disease and not for patients with relapsed or refractory disease. Also, the chance of relapsing after a mini-allogeneic transplant remains higher than after a full allogeneic transplant. This procedure should be considered only for relatively young patients and in general good health.

The chance of developing GVHD after nonmyeloablative transplant is still very significant. Therefore for the moment, mini-allogeneic transplants should be performed only as part of a clinical trial. The Bone Marrow Transplant Clinical Trials Network (BMT CTN) in the United States conducted a study to compare tandem autologous stem cell transplants versus a single autologous transplant followed by matched sibling nonmyeloblative allogeneic stem cell transplant. The results of this study indicated no benefit of the autologous transplant followed by the matched sibling nonmyeloblative allogeneic stem cell transplant, when compared to tandem autologous transplant, with respect to overall survival and progression-free survival in standard-risk[22] patients (CTN 0102 trial). This study and other similar studies will help physicians to determine if this approach is valid for treatment of myeloma. Also extremely important will be the results of studies designed to enhance the effect of the donor immune system after transplant. Mini-allogeneic transplant are performed on an outpatient basis; however, patients need to stay close to the treatment center for approximately the same time as patients undergoing a full-allogeneic transplant.

---

22 Standard-risk disease classification is the result of genetic interpretations of a patient's myeloma cells revealing no abnormalities associated with higher risk disease.

Syngeneic Transplant

In *syngeneic transplant*, the immune system of the donor is identical to the immune system of the recipient. In this type of transplant involving identical twins, the risk of GVHD is significantly lower. Thus, the risk of dying immediately after transplant and the potential side effects are very similar if not identical to an autologous transplant. The main advantage of a syngeneic transplant is that patients receive clean stem cells from a healthy donor. For this reason, patients who successfully complete a syngeneic transplant may live longer and also have a chance of being free of myeloma.

▶ Summary

Much remarkable progress has been made in the field of transplant for multiple myeloma. Currently, treatment with a short course of induction therapy followed by high-dose therapy and autologous stem cell transplant is the treatment of choice for many patients with multiple myeloma. Timing of transplant, the number of transplants, and the utility of maintenance therapy remain to be definitively determined. Both myeloablative and nonmyeloablative allogeneic transplant should be offered to younger patients only, and preferably in the context of a clinical trial. Finally, the introduction of the newer therapies has made an initially positive impact on the field of transplant and appear promising for the future.

CHAPTER 6

Supportive Care

S upportive care therapies are an important aspect of the treatment of a patient with multiple myeloma. These therapies can help patients cope with both complications due to the disease, and with the side effects of treatment. Ultimately, supportive care therapies can improve a patient's quality of life. Because myeloma is a disease of the immune system, its effects on the body can be widespread and varied. This chapter will discuss the role of supportive care to alleviate symptoms due to the myeloma including: anemia, fatigue, bone destruction, pain, elevated serum calcium, repeated infections, and numbness and tingling of the hands and feet due to peripheral neuropathy. This chapter will also briefly discuss the role of plasma exchange for treatment of hyperviscosity syndrome as well as the role of diet and exercise during treatment and recovery.

▶ Anemia

Anemia is one of the most common and debilitating complications of myeloma. Anemia may be mild (hemoglobin 10–11 g/dL), moderate (hemoglobin 10-8 g/dL), or severe (hemoglobin <8 g/dL). Anemia in myeloma is probably multifactorial, in newly diagnosed patients it is mainly due to inadequate erythropoietin (EPO) production related to the inflammatory cytokines like interleukin-1 and tumor necrosis factor. In the relapsed setting anemia can be a result of the atypical growth of malignant plasma cells in the bone marrow, leading in part to the suppression of red blood cell production, and/ or to a decreased production of erythropoietin in the kidneys due to immunoglobulin deposition damage from the myeloma. Some of the chemotherapy drugs used to treat myeloma can also cause anemia through their bone marrow suppressive (myelosuppressive) effects. Patients with anemia are usually tired and fatigued and they also may experience shortness of breath, rapid heartbeat, depression, insomnia, difficulty concentrating, and a pale appearance.

Treatment of Anemia

Anemia can be treated to improve the patient's quality of life. If a patient is experiencing symptoms due to moderate or severe anemia, he or she may need to be supported with red blood cell transfusions.[1] However, the benefit of blood transfusions is only temporary, as red blood cells live an average of 120 days and need to be replaced. Treatment with recombinant human erythropoietin (rhEPO)[2] and other erythroid-stimulating agents (ESAs)[3] improves anemia in patients with myeloma and severe kidney disease dialysis dependent, as they function to stimulate the production of red blood cells. Generally, EPO is injected under the skin (subcutaneously) and is given one to three times a week. Side effects of EPO are minor and include slight pain and/or irritation at the site of injection.

Darbepoietin (NESP) is a newer growth factor that also works by increasing the production of red blood cells and its mechanism of action is very similar to erythropoietin. Compared to EPO, NESP stays in the blood of a patient much longer, and can therefore be administered at less frequent intervals. There are concerns that using ESAs along with thalidomide, lenalidomide, and other immunomodulatory agents can increase the risk of thrombosis[4]

---

1 Blood cell transfusions refer to the process of giving various blood products into an individual's blood circulation intravenously.

2 Recombinant human erythropoietin (rhEPO) is an artificial hormone produced in cell culture that stimulates the production of red blood cells.

3 Erythroid-stimulating agents (ESAs) are medicines similar to erythropoietin that stimulate the production of red blood cells.

4 Thrombosis refers to blood clotting in a blood vessel, which can result in obstructed blood flow.

and there are some clinical studies showing worse outcomes in persons with a variety of cancers including myeloma, treated with ESAs compared to those who are not. This may be partly a result of an increase in blood thrombus as well as possible stimulation of cancer growth. Current recommendations for the use of ESAs can be found at the American Society of Hematology, the American Society of Clinical Oncology, and the National Comprehensive Cancer Network websites. Given the changing landscape regarding ESAs, it is important for each patient to have a discussion with his or her physician regarding the benefits and risks of ESA in his or her particular situation.

▶ Fatigue

Fatigue can be due to the underlying myeloma, anemia, poor nutrition, infection, and/or depression, and it can also be a side effect of chemotherapy or other therapies, including the medications used to control pain. The treatment of myeloma-induced fatigue can greatly improve a patient's quality of life. Fatigue will improve with the treatment of the underlying cause. For example, fatigue will improve by treating the myeloma with chemotherapy or other antimyeloma drugs, by treating the anemia, by treating infections with antibiotics and, if possible, by adjusting the dose of the medications that can possibly cause fatigue. Also, some patients may benefit from antidepressants, a physical exercise program, or nutrition counseling.

▶ Pain Management

Pain is experienced subjectively, and therefore it is important that the doctor and/or nursing staff obtain a pain history directly from the patient. Studies on pain have shown that pain is normally underestimated by healthcare providers and overestimated by family members. Patients are typically asked to describe the characteristics of pain such as: the location of the pain, the distribution, the quality, and the intensity. Physical and neurologic examinations are also very important components of the pain assessment. Pain assessment is an ongoing process and patients need to be assessed by the healthcare providers at regular intervals. Ultimately, the management of pain includes selection of the appropriate drugs, dose adjustments, relief of breakthrough pain, and management of side effects.

The World Health Organization (WHO) provides a three-step analgesic ladder to choose the type of medication based on the severity of the pain. Step 1 of the WHO ladder includes nonopioid analgesics for mild pain (1 to 3 on a 10-point scale), step 2 includes low-dose opioids for moderate pain and nonopioids plus adjuvants (4 to 6), and step 3 includes high-dose opioids and nonopioids plus adjuvants and is reserved only for severe pain (7 to 10).

Opioids[5] are associated with many side effects including constipation, nausea, vomiting, and sedation. True allergy to an opioid is rare. Adjuvant agents[6] (coanalgesics) are sometimes used in combination with an opioid because they can provide relief in specific situations, especially if the pain is due to a nerve impingement. Adjuvant agents include: steroids, antiseizure medications, antidepressants, and local anesthetics.

Alternative methods for pain relief can be acupuncture and yoga. Because nonsteroidal anti-inflammatory drugs (NSAIDs)[7] may cause kidney damage, and kidney damage is a common consequence of myeloma, your doctor may recommend that you avoid taking them. Aspirin, a NSAID, can cause problems with blood clotting by interfering with platelets so it may have to be avoided when the myeloma or treatment causes low platelet counts. In general, it is very important to check every medication taken (including over-the-counter or alternative medications) with the physician, as they may all have serious side effects in people with myeloma. For difficult to manage pain, consultation with a specialist in pain management can be particularly helpful as well as important.

---

5 Opioids are a class of medications that relieve pain.
6 Adjuvant agents (coanalgesics) are therapies given alongside a primary therapy in order to maximize its effectiveness.
7 Nonsteroidal anti-inflammatory drugs (NSAIDs) are a class of drugs used to reduce inflammation, pain, and fever.

▶ Bone Destruction

Bone destruction in multiple myeloma is due to an increased number and activity of osteoclasts, as well as a decrease in number and activity of osteoblasts (see Chapter 2). Osteoclasts grow in the vicinity of myeloma cells and myeloma cells produce substances that enhance their activity (IL-1, TNF, and M-CSF). More recently, it was discovered that in patients with myeloma there is an imbalance between two important substances, RANKL and OPG; this imbalance also contributes greatly to the bone loss observed in myeloma. Patients with moderate to severe bone destruction will present with bone pain, elevated serum calcium levels, and bone fractures. Collapsed vertebrae can lead to nerve impingement, spinal cord compression, and a decrease in height. Treatment of bone destruction includes management of the bone pain and elevated calcium, management of the bone fractures with local radiotherapy, and sometimes, surgical stabilization and treatment with bisphosphonate therapy (see below).

▶ Treatment of Elevated Calcium (Hypercalcemia)

Hypercalcemia is a disorder in which the level of calcium in the blood is too high. Healthy individuals maintain equilibrium between ingested calcium from diet and lost calcium through urine. In patients with myeloma this equilibrium is disrupted because there is an increase in the amount of calcium due to the bone loss and a decreased ability of the kidneys to excrete the excess of free calcium. The most common symptoms of hypercalcemia are fatigue, lack of appetite, tiredness, nausea, vomiting, constipation, frequent urination, increased thirst, lethargy, and difficulty thinking clearly. Other common symptoms are depression, indifference, confusion, and restlessness. Some patients may experience only few symptoms and others may have not symptoms at all. Treatment of the underlying myeloma is the best therapy for myeloma-associated hypercalcemia. Patients presenting with mild hypercalcemia and no symptoms may be treated with fluids given by vein and require close observation while receiving appropriate antimyeloma treatment. Patients presenting with more severe hypercalcemia require immediate initiation of drugs to lower the calcium level, such as calcitonin[8] and bisphosphonates. Dialysis is used to treat patients with increased calcium and kidney failure. Patients and family members should be aware of the symptoms of hypercalcemia, because if not treated appropriately, it can be a life-threatening condition.

▶ Bisphosphonate Therapy

Bisphosphonate therapy is recommended for all patients with evidence of bone destruction due to the myeloma. Bisphosphonates are a class of drugs analogous to naturally produced chemicals that function by binding to calcium crystals. After subsequent release and uptake by osteoclasts, they prevent bone reabsorption by inhibiting osteoclasts from growing and causing bone damage. They also block the production of interleukin-6 (IL-6) and therefore they also directly work against the myeloma cells. Several large studies showed that patients receiving biphosphonate every month experienced a lower number of new bone lesions and bone fractures compared to patients that did not. Bisphosphonates also help to control the pain due to bone destruction.

The two most commonly used bisphosphonate drugs in myeloma are pamidronate (Aredia©) and zoledronic acid (Zometa©). They are both administered intravenously because they are not well absorbed when given by mouth. Pamidronate is given at a dose of 90 mg and it is infused over a couple of hours every 3 to 4 weeks. Zoledronic acid is much more potent than pamidronate, so the dose given is lower (4 mg), and it is infused over 15 minutes every 3 to 4 weeks. Recent studies and a randomized trial have shown that the use of zoledronic acid once every 12 weeks compared with the standard dosing interval of once every 4 weeks is equally effective at preventing the onset of skeletal events. The longer dosing interval may eventually become the standard of care option.

---

8 Calcitonin is a hormone that helps regulate calcium and phosphate levels in the bloodstream.

The main side effects of biphosphonates are fever (typically occurring within the first 24 hours of administration), fatigue, weakness, and renal damage. A less common but quite concerning side effect of these drugs is osteonecrosis of the jaw (ONJ).[9] The reason the bones of the jaw are more often affected than other bones in the body is probably in part, related to the antiangiogenic side effects of bisphosphonates. Injury to the jaw via tooth extraction, dental surgery, or microfracture can lead to osteonecrosis as a result of improper or suppressed remodeling mechanisms resulting from the bisphosphonate therapy.

Patients taking bisphosphonate drugs should be advised to maintain good oral hygiene and see their dentist periodically for cleaning and general evaluation. Additionally, it is not recommended to undergo any dental procedures, such as a tooth extraction, while taking these drugs. If necessary, the dentist or oral surgeon should be aware that the patient is taking bisphosphonate therapy and that the risk of developing this condition is elevated. Patients on bisphosphonate therapy should notify their physician immediately if they experience tooth or jaw pain, numbness, or have any evidence of mouth sores. The treatment of the osteonecrosis of the jaw is difficult and currently not very effective, so preventive measures are important. All patients, prior to receiving bisphosphonate therapy, should be educated about ONJ and should undergo proper dental evaluation. Smoking can also increase the risk of osteonecrosis of the jaw and therefore a smoking cessation program should be considered prior to initiation of therapy. It is important to understand that while this complication is a possible risk, it is not common, and the risk is outweighed by the benefits obtained by this therapy. In fact, studies conducted to assess the benefit of these drugs showed that bisphosphonate therapy reduced the number of bone destructive lesions and thereby improved the quality of life of patients with myeloma.

---

9 Osteonecrosis of the jaw (ONJ) is a condition that occurs when the jawbone becomes exposed and begins to degenerate as a result of inadequate blood supply.

▶ RANK Ligand (RANKL) Inhibition

Denosumab (XGEVA©) is a human IgG monoclonal antibody that was approved by the FDA in 2010 for the treatment of bone metastases from solid tumors, though it has yet to obtain approval for use in multiple myeloma. It functions by binding to cytokine RANKL, which is an essential molecule in initiating bone turnover. By inhibiting RANKL, denosumab blocks osteoclast maturation, function, and survival. This ultimately results in a reduction of bone loss. This mechanism of action lies in contrast to bisphosphonates, which bind bone mineral and are absorbed by osteoclasts that subsequently undergo cell death.

A phase III study of 1718 patients compared denosumab with zoledronic acid in the prevention of skeletal-related events in adult patients with newly diagnosed multiple myeloma and bone disease. In this study denosumab was found to be noninferior to zoledronic acid at delaying the time to first skeletal-related event for patients with multiple myeloma. Additionally, denosumab is not cleared by the kidneys and may offer a safe and effective option for patients with renal impairment. The dosage of denosumab in the large phase III study conducted in multiple myeloma was 120 mg given subcutaneously every 4 weeks.

Side effects of denosumab include fatigue, low phosphate levels in the blood, nausea, and hypocalcemia. Since over 90% of patients with MM develop osteolytic lesions during the course of the disease, preventing bone complications is an important aspect of caring for patients with MM. Skeletal events can cause significant morbidity and negatively impact patient quality of life. Important research is ongoing to develop additional therapies that help restore the body's natural bone remolding process in order to prevent bone loss and fractures in patients with multiple myeloma.

▶ Treatment of Bone Fractures

Approximately 30% of patients will have their multiple myeloma first discovered when they develop a pathologic fracture. The spine is the most common location for a myeloma destructive lesion. Other common locations are the ribs and the bones of the pelvis.

Pathologic fractures of non–weight-bearing bones can be safely treated with radiotherapy. In contrast, surgical intervention should be considered to treat pathologic fractures of long bones of the arms and legs. Surgical intervention and radiotherapy can be also used to prevent the occurrence of a pathologic fracture for those lesions that are considered at high risk. While the incidence of long bone fractures is relatively low, pathologic fractures of the vertebral bodies are very common in myeloma patients.

Vertebral body fractures are associated with severe pain and height loss. The pain can be severe and may last for many months. Pain often is not well controlled with medical management or antimyeloma treatment. Patients experiencing back pain due to pathologic fracture should be referred to a specialist orthopedist or interventional radiology with experience in modern spinal intervention. Vertebroplasty is a minimally invasive surgery that involves the injection of a cement-like substance into the vertebral body to stabilize the fracture. It is performed in an outpatient facility under local anesthesia. Side effects associated with the procedure are minimal. In rare instances however, the filler substance may leak out and cause pain. Also, with this procedure the height of the vertebral body is not restored.

Kyphoplasty is a newer technique developed to overcome some of the drawbacks of vertebroplasty and is now more commonly used. Kyphoplasty can restore some height of the compressed vertebrae. The procedure can be performed in an outpatient facility under local anesthesia. It involves making a small incision in the back and inserting an inflatable balloon into the compressed vertebrae. The inflated balloon creates a cavity that can be then filled with a cement-like substance. On average, 30%–40% of the height lost can be restored. The side effects associated with kyphoplasty are minimal. These procedures have significant beneficial impact on the quality of life of patients with myeloma.

Compression of the spinal cord or instability of the spinal cord due to a vertebral body fracture occurs in 10%–20% of patients. In addition to complaining of back pain, patients with compression of the spinal cord may also experience weakness and numbness or paralysis of arms and/or legs. Suspected compression of the spinal cord is a medical emergency and requires immediate evaluation by a physician. Normally, spinal MRI is the test of choice to make a diagnosis of spinal cord compression although CT scans can sometimes also be helpful. Standard X-rays of the spine are typically not useful in diagnosing spinal cord compression. Treatment generally includes prompt initiation of high-dose steroids (dexamethasone 16 mg/day in divided doses) and immediate referral for radiotherapy or surgery. Surgery is normally indicated if there is evidence of spinal cord instability. After surgical stabilization of a pathologic fracture or radiotherapy, patients can initiate a rehabilitation program. Careful, tailored exercise is important to help maintain function, quality of life, and to gently enhance the noncancerous portions of the bone.

▶ Peripheral Neuropathy

Peripheral neuropathy is a disorder of the peripheral nervous system. The peripheral nervous system includes all nerves outside the brain and the spinal cord, encompassing all nerves of the face, arms, legs, torso, and some nerves in the skull. The nerves provide a communication between the brain and the rest of the body; when the nerves are damaged this communication is altered or interrupted. The most common symptoms of peripheral neuropathy are: sharp or burning pain, tingling sensation, abnormal or altered sensation to touch, numbness, weakness, tremor, and muscle cramps. Some patients also complain of lack of coordination performing simple tasks. For example, buttoning a shirt may be very difficult. In myeloma, the nerves that are most commonly affected are those of the hands and feet.

Causes of Peripheral Neuropathy

The most common causes of peripheral neuropathy in patients with myeloma are side effects of medications such as vincristine, carboplatinum, thalidomide, and bortezomib (Velcade©). Sometimes the excess production of myeloma protein can cause the blood to be more viscous, causing poor circulation, which can lead to peripheral neuropathy. The paraprotein can also cause direct damaging of the nerves by depositing on the nerve tissue. Peripheral neuropathy is not very common in patients with newly diagnosed multiple myeloma, but is more common in patients with AL amyloidosis, Waldenstrom macroglobulinemia, in patients with kidney damage, and in patients with MGUS (monoclonal gammopathy of undetermined significance). About one-third of patients with MGUS have symptoms of peripheral neuropathy. The IgM class is the most common paraprotein associated with peripheral neuropathy in patients with MGUS (60%), followed by IgG (30%) and IgA (10%). Approximately half of patients with IgM MGUS have antibodies that bind to the nerve myelin[10] or anti-MAG antibodies (myelin-associated glycoprotein). Biopsy of the peripheral nerve is important to identify the anti-MAG myelin antibodies and also to detect the deposition of the protein in the nerve tissue occurring in patients with amyloidosis and in patients with light-chain deposition disease.[11]

Treatment of Peripheral Neuropathy

The main treatment of peripheral neuropathy is eliminating or reducing the primary cause. For example, if the cause of the neuropathy is the myeloma itself, then treating the myeloma will reduce the symptoms. If the peripheral neuropathy is caused by a medication, then discontinuing the drug for a period of time or lowering the dose may help alleviate the symptoms. Sometimes the pain caused by peripheral neuropathy can be controlled using antidepressant drugs or antiepileptic drugs. Other treatments may include pain medications such as opioid drugs, local anesthetic injections, and supplements with vitamin B complex, folic acid, and magnesium tablets. A transcutaneous electrical nerve stimulation (TENS) machine can also be used to alleviate the pain caused by the peripheral neuropathy. The machine works by sending small electrical impulses to the nerve using small electrodes placed on the skin of the patient. Some patients might find some relief from simple

---

10 Myelin is a fatty substance that coats nerve fibers and functions to increase the speed of electrical communication in the nervous system.
11 Light-chain deposition disease (LCDD) is a plasma cell disorder involving the deposition of the light-chain portion of immunoglobulins into organ systems, most often the kidneys. This condition is a distinct entity from amyloidosis and multiple myeloma. Also termed *light-chain disease.*

relaxation techniques, massage, and acupuncture. Regular gentle exercise can help to keep muscles toned and to improve circulation, thus helping to mitigate the effects of peripheral neuropathy.

▶ Infections

Infections are frequent complications of patients with multiple myeloma. In patients with early-stage myeloma, the most common infections involve the respiratory tract, manifesting as bronchitis and pneumonia. In patients with advanced stage myeloma, infections of the blood and urinary tract infections are more common.

Prevention of Infections

All patients with multiple myeloma, in particular patients with advanced myeloma or patients receiving chemotherapy, should be instructed to contact their physician immediately at the first sign of infection. For patients with a history of recurrent infections, a large study has shown that the administration of monthly immunoglobulin intravenously (IVIg)[12] for a period of 1 year reduces both the frequency and the severity of infections. Unfortunately, intravenous immunoglobulin is not a benign therapy and should be used only in selected patients. Infusion-related side effects may include chills, headaches, nausea, vomiting, and dizziness. Severe adverse reactions may include hemolytic anemia,[13] anaphylaxis, and renal failure among others. Antibiotics such as prophylaxis[14] given by mouth are also used to reduce the incidence of infection in patients receiving chemotherapy; however, the data regarding this are limited. Patients on high-dose steroids should receive concomitant treatment to prevent fungal infection of the gastrointestinal tract and to prevent herpes infections. Steroids can cause increased

---

12 Intravenous immunoglobulin (IVIg) is an immunomodulatory agent given intravenously in patients with suppressed immune systems to help prevent infection.
13 Hemolytic anemia is a type of anemia that results from the abnormal breakdown of red blood cells.
14 Prophylaxis refers to a measure, such as an antibiotic, taken to prevent a disease or infection.

glucose levels in the blood, providing an environment for potentially increased fungal proliferation. Patients receiving proteasome inhibitors combined with steroids or other chemotherapy agents have a high risk (25%) of developing herpetic infections and should also receive prophylactic treatment[15] with antiviral drugs.

Treatment of Infections

Developing an infection when someone has a low white blood cell count, is receiving treatment for myeloma, or has advanced myeloma, is a medical emergency. Patients who develop fever or other symptoms should be seen by a physician immediately. If infection is suspected, patients with low blood counts should promptly receive a course of broad-spectrum antibiotics intravenously. G-CSF (Neupogen) is routinely used together with antibiotics to speed up the white blood cells recovery after transplant and/or after intravenous chemotherapy.

▶ Hyperviscosity Syndrome

In addition to bone pain, fatigue due to anemia, and recurrent infections due to suppression of the normal immune system, patients with multiple myeloma can present with other symptoms due to the excessive production of the atypical protein or immunoglobulin in the blood. When the abnormal protein reaches a high concentration in the blood, it can cause the blood to become more viscous. Symptoms due to thick blood, or *hyperviscosity syndrome*, include chest pain, shortness of breath, confusion, dizziness, fatigue, drowsiness, vertigo, blurred vision, and sometimes bleeding.

Hyperviscosity syndrome is a rare complication of multiple myeloma. It occurs more often in patients with immunocytoma (Waldenstrom's macroglobulinemia, an IgM disorder) and less frequently in patients with IgA or IgG3 multiple myeloma types. Hyperviscosity syndrome is a medical emergency and patients with symptoms of thick blood require immediate intervention. Because

---

15 Prophylactic treatment refers to the prevention of potential complications resulting from infection with the use of antibiotics.

it may take up to several days or even weeks for the treatment of the underlying myeloma to start working, patients with severe symptoms due to thick blood may require treatment with plasmapheresis or plasma exchange.

Plasmapheresis is a procedure used to remove the excess M-protein and/or other substances. A cell separator is used to separate the fluid part of the blood, called plasma, from the blood cells. In the separator machine, the blood is spun at high speed and in this way the cells are separated from the plasma. Another way to separate the blood cells from the plasma is by passing the blood through a filter. The plasma is discarded and replaced with plasma of a healthy individual and then the cells and the healthy plasma are returned to the patient through a small catheter placed into a vein. Often a medication to prevent the blood from clotting when it is outside the body is given to the patient during this procedure. During plasma exchange, some patients might experience a drop in their blood pressure. Because of this possibility, they should talk with their doctor about temporarily holding their blood pressure medications.

Other minor common side effects that patients can experience during or after this procedure include tingling or numbness around the mouth or in the arms or legs, muscle cramps, dizziness, nausea, and lightheadedness. Also, because some drugs are removed from the blood during plasma exchange, some medications dosage adjustment may be necessary until the procedure is completed. Plasmapheresis is an effective treatment; however, it is only a temporary measure. Patients with symptoms due to hyperviscocity syndrome are encouraged to remain well hydrated.

▶ Role of Diet and Exercise

A healthy balanced diet includes a variety of foods such as fruit, vegetables, foods high in fiber, good sources of protein such as fish and chicken, limited red or processed meat, and few fried foods. A well-balanced diet may help increase energy and aid in recovery. Maintaining an adequate fluid intake is also important to mitigate kidney damage and symptoms of hyperviscocity syndrome. Patients receiving bisphosphonate therapy should maintain an adequate calcium intake. Exercise and an active lifestyle not only control weight, but can also influence hormone levels and the immune system function. Regular gentle exercise can help keep the bones relatively strong, reduce fatigue, and help with depression as well as improve sleep. In a study conducted to examine the association between exercise and quality of life in multiple myeloma, patients who exercised regularly both during and while off treatment reported a higher quality of life.

▶ Summary

Learning to manage the various symptoms associated with multiple myeloma is essential to maintain quality of life for a patient. Understanding the treatments for multiple myeloma and their side effects is also important. Asking questions, effectively making important decisions, maintaining an active support group, and setting goals can help patients cope with this challenging disease. Finally, eating well and exercising regularly should be made a priority as they can significantly enhance patient quality of life.

CHAPTER 7

Searching for the Cure

▶ Introduction

There has been a dramatic increase in the number and type of promising new agents including targeted drugs, antibodies, and vaccines that have been developed for treating multiple myeloma in the last several years. Many of these new treatments have been developed based on an improved understanding of the biology of myeloma and how it grows and spreads within the body. This has allowed for the development of agents that attack specific targets in the myeloma cells as compared to classic chemotherapy, which broadly kills many cell types. New agents are initially tested in the laboratory then in phase I, II, and III clinical trials (see Chapter 4). If the new agent is found to be useful with reasonable side effects, it may be approved by the FDA and subsequently prescribed by a doctor like any other approved medicine. Until approval occurs, many new agents are available to patients who enroll in clinical trials.

In this chapter, we will discuss some of the new classes of agents that are being tested as well as the basis for their development. It is important to remember that new agents are continuously being developed and rejected because many are found to be either ineffective or too toxic. Consequently, the list of new agents is constantly changing. The Multiple Myeloma Research Foundation (MMRF) maintains a website at www.themmrf.org/multiple-myeloma-knowledge-center /experimental-treatments/ and the International Myeloma Foundation (IMF) has a website called "The Myeloma Matrix" at http://myeloma .org/matrix that keeps an updated list of emerging therapies. Additional information on available clinical trials can be found at the MMRF at

www.multiplemyeloma.org/clinical_trials, the IMF at www.myeloma
.org, or at the National Institute of Cancer website at www.cancer.gov
/clinicaltrials. The following is a brief summary of some of the
newer and emerging broad classes of therapies that may ultimately
play important roles in the treatment of myeloma. Drugs that are
currently being tested and evaluated can be found via the websites
previously mentioned above.

▶ Angiogenesis Inhibitors

An interesting finding is that myeloma growth is dependent on the
growth of new blood vessels into the area where the disease spreads.
This process, called angiogenesis, was known for years to be important
in solid tumors like breast cancer and colon cancer but was somewhat
unexpected in a nonsolid cancer like myeloma. It is now thought
that at least some of the activity of thalidomide, lenalidomide, and
pomalidomide functions through blocking angiogenesis. Another
interesting finding is that myeloma cells themselves express some
important growth proteins that are normally found on the cells that
line blood vessels (endothelial cells). One of the most important
of these is vascular endothelial growth factor receptor (VEGFR),
which responds to a hormone called vascular endothelial growth
factor (VEGF) to promote cell growth (see Chapter 2). A number
of agents that attack the VEGFR or VEGF have been developed
and are currently in various stages of testing. Another approach is
to use genetically engineered monoclonal antibodies to block the
simulation of VEGFR by VEGF. While effective inhibition of tumor
angiogenesis helps to halt tumor progression, it would likely not
eliminate the tumor alone. Therefore it may be essential for agents
that inhibit angiogenesis be paired with other treatments for effective cancer eradication.

▶ Inhibitors of Myeloma Growth Processes

All cells, including myeloma cells, respond to signals in their environment through a series of networks called signaling pathways.
Depending on which signaling pathways are activated, a cell may

be stimulated to divide, stop growing, mature, or die. For example, when VEGF binds to the VEGFR on the surface of a myeloma cell, a signal is sent through a series of signaling pathways to the DNA in the nucleus of the cell, where a number of genes get turned on which drive the myeloma cell to divide. Based on this phenomenon, many researchers are trying to define how the signaling pathways work in myeloma cells and then design medications that can either block or activate various parts of the pathways.

One important pathway is called the phosphatidylinositol-3 kinase pathway (or PI3K pathway). A key part of the PIK3 pathway is a protein called Akt[1], so this pathway is also frequently called the PI3K/Akt pathway. Many of the most important myeloma growth factors, including IL-6, VEGF, and IGF-1, bind to receptors on the surface of myeloma cells called tyrosine kinase receptors[2] and subsequently trigger the PI3K/Akt pathway. Because of its importance in the growth and survival of myeloma cells, a number of drugs are being developed and tested to block the PI3K/Akt pathway. mTOR (mammalian target of rapamycin) is a key protein involved in the growth and spread of myeloma cells. Several drugs have been developed that target mTOR. These drugs have been shown to block the growth of myeloma cells in the laboratory. Another important signaling pathway in myeloma is called the mitogen-activated protein kinase (MAPK) pathway. One of the members of this pathway is a protein termed Ras.[3] This protein must be modified in order for it to work by an enzyme termed farnesyltransferase. Several farnesyltransferase inhibitor (FTIs) drugs have been developed. The FTIs have been shown in the laboratory to block the growth of myeloma cells and appear to work to increase the activity of bortezomib. C-Jun

---

1 Akt, also called protein kinase B (PKB), is a protein that plays a key role in multiple cellular processes including cell migration, metabolism, proliferation, and apoptosis.
2 Tyrosine kinase receptors are cell surface receptors for many cytokines, hormones, and growth factors.
3 Ras is a family of related proteins involved in the signals passed between cells that regulate the amount of growth allowed at any given time. Mutations of the gene that encodes Ras can result in a form of the protein that promotes cancer growth.

N-terminal protein kinase (JNK) is another protein kinase[4] and member of the MAPK pathway. When it is inactivated, myeloma cells appear to be protected from some forms of apoptosis. Consequently, researchers have been developing drugs that activate (rather than block) JNK so that drugs that cause myeloma cell apoptosis can be more effective.

Nuclear factor κB (NF-κB) is another key member of the pathways that are important in myeloma cell growth and survival and plays a role in angiogenesis as well. Because NF-κB is dysregulated in myeloma, a number of drugs have been developed to try to block it. Thalidomide, dexamethasone, bortezomib, and arsenic work at least in part, by inhibition of NF-κB. Newer agents that inhibit NF-κB are being tested in the laboratory will likely eventually make their way into clinical trials.

Cyclin-dependent kinases (CDKs) are protein kinases that play a central role in regulation of the cell cycle. Dysregulation of CDKs is a hallmark of multiple myeloma. Small molecule drugs[5] that function to inhibit CDKs are currently being developed and tested. Some types of CDK inhibition has been shown to enhance the activity of proteasome inhibitors, suggesting that combining these two drugs may be able to synergize to produce an enhanced effect.

Kinesin spindle protein (KSP) is a motor protein that plays a critical role in cells that are undergoing division. Targeted inhibition of this protein blocks cell division and causes dividing myeloma cells to undergo programmed cell death (apoptosis) by depleting mcl-1 (see below). KSP inhibition represents a novel approach to treating multiple myeloma and drugs that facilitate this may be active in myeloma cells that are resistant to proteasome inhibitors and immunomodulatory drugs due to its novel mechanism of action.

The nucleus of a cell contains specific tumor-suppressor proteins that function to protect the cell against malignant transformation. In multiple myeloma, these proteins are transported out of the

---

4 Protein kinase refers to an enzyme that modifies other proteins, causing a functional change in the targeted protein.
5 Small molecule drugs are very low-weight organic compounds that can cross cell membranes. Most pharmaceutical drugs are small molecules.

myeloma cell nucleus in large numbers, and are therefore unable to act against the progression of cancer. Transporter proteins such as XPO1[6] help to regulate the transport of proteins outside the nucleus. Research has shown that myeloma cells overproduce nuclear transporter proteins like XPO1, causing several essential proteins including tumor suppressor proteins to be exported out of the nucleus, thereby aiding in cancer progression. Targeting overproduced transporter proteins like XPO1 via small molecule inhibition represents a promising approach to treat multiple myeloma.

▶ Agents that Affect Apoptosis

All the cells in the body are programmed to live for only a certain amount of time and then to die in an orderly process called programmed cell death, or apoptosis. One way that cancer develops is that cells lose their ability to undergo the normal apoptosis process. When this happens, the cells accumulate instead of doing their job and then dying off, as should normally happen. Many myeloma cells are able to survive and continue to reproduce because they produce higher levels of a protein called Bcl-2[7] and other related proteins that block the normal process of apoptosis. The effects of Bcl-2 and related proteins may also prevent many drugs like dexamethasone from working because many drugs work by triggering apoptosis in the myeloma cells. Blocking Bcl-2 and other related proteins restores the ability to undergo cellular apoptosis and could help make drugs like dexamethasone work better. All cells make proteins like Bcl-2 by first producing a coding molecule termed messenger RNA (mRNA)[8] from the DNA, which directs the assembly of the protein by a molecular factory inside the cell called a ribosome.[9]

---

6 XPO1, or exportin 1, is a protein that mediates the export of proteins and other functional products out of the cell nucleus.

7 Bcl-2, or B-cell lymphoma 2, is the founding member of a family of proteins involved in regulating cell death.

8 mRNA, or messenger RNA, refers to a large family of molecules that convey genetic information from the DNA to the site of protein production.

9 Ribosome is a complex molecule that functions as a molecular factory for protein synthesis in the cell.

An antisense molecule is an RNA or similar molecule that can bind to the mRNA and cause it to be blocked or destroyed. This results in reduced production of the protein coded for by the mRNA. In the case of Bcl-2, blocking its production by treating myeloma cells with antisense molecules causes the cells to undergo apoptosis, particularly when they are exposed to other drugs such as dexamethasone.

In addition to antisense, other types of drugs are being developed that bind to and inactivate the Bcl-2 protein. Antisense and drugs are also being developed to target other proteins that are related to Bcl-2, including proteins called Bcl-B and Mcl-1, as there is some evidence that they may be more important in governing apoptosis in myeloma cells than Bcl-2. Ultimately, this strategy of attacking targets like Bcl-2 that keep myeloma cells from dying may be helpful in the treatment of myeloma, particularly when combined with other medications.

▶ Immune Therapies and Vaccinations

As described in Chapter 2, antibodies are proteins naturally produced by plasma cells and B cells. In the last two decades, genetic engineering techniques have been developed that allow researchers to tailor make therapeutic antibodies directed against specific targets. This approach has proven very successful for certain types of lymphoma. Therapeutic antibodies contribute to improved treatment outcomes and therefore have become part of the standard of care for these diseases. In the case of myeloma, researchers have been working to identify targets on the myeloma cells and then genetically engineering antibodies that would attack these targets, thereby destroying the myeloma cells as well. There are many proteins on the surface of myeloma cells that may serve as targets for therapeutic antibodies. Targets on the surface of myeloma cells for which antibodies have been developed include proteins called CD20, CD138, CD40, CD56, FGFR3, EGFR, IL-6, and its receptor, and PD-L1 (see below).

As described in Chapter 2, the role of the immune system is to protect the body from foreign invaders. Normally, the immune system responds to tumor cells by eliminating them as they would a foreign substance. T cells play a central role in this immune response and are activated by antigen-presenting cells called dendritic cells[10] in the lymph nodes. They then make their way into the tumor microenvironment where the now-activated T cells work to destroy the cancer cells. There are a number of proteins on T cells that serve as *checkpoints*, allowing them to be turned on and off as needed. Tumor cells can exploit these checkpoints to "turn off" immune responses and, therefore, prevent cancer cell death.

PD-L1 is an inhibitory ligand that, in normal conditions, helps to maintain immune homeostasis. Recent evidence shows that in multiple myeloma, PD-L1 helps myeloma cells evade the immune system. By binding to its receptors B7.1 and PD-1 that are expressed on the surface of activated T cells, PD-L1 causes the inactivation of these T cells. Research has shown that expression of PD-L1 is upregulated in multiple myeloma and functions as an important suppressor of effective anticancer immune responses in many patients. Significant progress is underway to develop drugs that inhibit "checkpoints" like the PD-1/PD-L1 pathway. These drugs will likely be used in combination with other myeloma treatments to produce a more pronounced effect.

Chimeric antigen-receptor T-cell (CAR-T) therapy refers to a type of treatment in which a patient's T cells are removed from their blood and reengineered to target and bind to a certain protein antigen expressed on the patient's cancer cells. These CAR-T cells are then grown in large quantities in the laboratory and reintroduced intravenously into the patient's bloodstream. After the CAR-T cells are introduced back into the patient, they multiply, recognize, and kill cancer cells harboring the antigen for which they were designed to eliminate. Significant research is being devoted to optimize this therapy as well as to determine optimal cellular antigen targets. Cell surface markers including CD19 and BCMA,[11] among others, have been identified as targets for CAR-T therapy in patients with multiple myeloma.

---

10 Dendritic cells are immune cells that function to process antigen material and present it on their cell surfaces to prime immune system T cells.
11 BCMA, or B-cell maturation antigen, is a protein that plays a key role in B-cell development and autoimmune responses.

Vaccines are substances used to provide immunity against diseases and function by stimulating the production of antibodies. Vaccines that are designed to treat a disease rather than prevent it are termed *therapeutic vaccines*. Anticancer vaccines are designed to activate the body's immune response against cancer cells in a similar fashion to how vaccines are traditionally used to promote immune defenses against infection. A number of efforts over the past several years have been made to develop a therapeutic vaccine against myeloma. The long-term hope with this strategy is that after a patient has achieved a remission with other drugs, the vaccine therapy would be introduced with the purpose of maintaining the patient's remission for an extended period of time, given that the individual's immune system is functioning adequately. Research has shown that immune system targets in multiple myeloma tend to be stable over time, even as resistance to therapies targeting mutated cell surface antigens and signaling pathways develops, thus highlighting the potential efficacy of this therapy.

Many therapeutic vaccine[12] studies have chosen the idiotype protein, the specific immunoglobulin produced by the individual's myeloma, as the antigen used to stimulate an immune response. One advantage of using the idiotype protein to stimulate an immune response is that only the myeloma cells make this protein so the immune response to the vaccine may only be directed against the myeloma cells rather than against normal tissues. While laboratory evidence of an immune response to the idiotype protein has been observed in many vaccinated persons, significant and long-lasting effects against the myeloma have not been routinely observed. Because of this, researchers have been trying to develop more potent vaccines. One approach to boosting the action of the vaccine is to couple it with vaccination with a type of cell called a dendritic cell. Because the normal job of dendritic cells is to turn on the immune system in response to infections and other problems, these dendritic cell/idiotype protein vaccines may stimulate the immune system

12 Therapeutic vaccines are vaccines that are not used as a preventative measure, but rather, as a method of treatment. Therapeutic vaccines function by stimulating the immune system to target a type of diseased cell or infection.

more than when the idiotype protein is used alone in the vaccine. Additional research is being conducted to determine if other myeloma-associated antigens could more potently stimulate the immune system and whether other types of treatment could further amplify the immune response to the vaccine.

Virotherapy is an emerging treatment modality that is based around modifying and reprogramming viruses to attack cancer cells while sparing normal tissues. These oncolytic viruses[13] are designed to selectively infect and lead do the destruction of cancer cells, while leaving normal cells and tissue relatively unharmed. Several oncolytic viruses have been investigated including reengineered measles virus and reovirus. Ideally the goal of this therapy, like others, would be to provide a long treatment-free remission period for patients. The results of clinical trials and future studies regarding this form of therapy are awaited with interest.

▶ Personalized Medicine

Mounting evidence supports the idea that every case of cancer is unique. Patient characteristics including environmental factors, other medical conditions, family history, genetic mutations, and myeloma disease features all factor into each patient's presentation, response to treatment, and overall outcome. Therefore, we can consider each case of cancer, and therefore each case of myeloma, to be distinct in each patient. The goal of personalized medicine is to create targeted therapies that work in key patient populations based on specific genetic features. As described in Chapter 2, multiple myeloma is characterized by genetic mutations that affect gene activity and expression. These genetic mutations alongside each individual's genetic makeup can be thought of as fingerprints that provide a unique profile of behavior for each patient's myeloma. Efforts are underway to build a future in which a personalized treatment plan can be created based on the characteristics and behavior of an individual's myeloma.

---

13 Oncolytic virus refers to a virus that infects and destroys cancer cells. The destroyed cancer cells release new infectious viruses, which help destroy additional cancer cells.

By using techniques such as genomic sequencing[14] and gene expression profiling (GEP), physicians and researchers are working to identify genetic markers in each patient's disease that can be targeted with specific treatments. Advances in computational biology and studies on large patient populations are also beginning to allow researchers to predict whether or not a given treatment may be effective nor not based on a patient's own genetic profile.

▶ Summary

This chapter has summarized just a fraction of the emerging treatment strategies that are under development, in hopes of illustrating a few examples of the approaches that are being taken to develop new treatments for myeloma. Novel versions of established therapies including new alkylating agents, new proteasome inhibitors, new immunomodulatory agents, and new monoclonal antibodies are being developed and tested for use.

However, the future of myeloma treatment may be to expand even further beyond these established modalities. Identifying the most effective and best-tolerated combinations of the emerging therapies will be particularly challenging and exciting. As more is understood about how myeloma develops, grows, and becomes resistant to existing agents, even more progress will be made in the development of novel generations of treatments. In addition, there are a multitude of research studies and clinical trials underway to improve the diagnosis of myeloma, reduce bone disease, and improve supportive care and quality of life. The enormous number of potentially useful new agents raises great hope that progress will continue to be made in the treatment of multiple myeloma. It is not too far-fetched to predict that one or more of these emerging therapies will help turn myeloma more into the likes of a manageable chronic disease and furthermore, ultimately help lead to a cure.

---

14 Genomic sequencing refers to the process of determining the complete DNA sequence of an individual's genetic material.

Index

Note: Page numbers followed by *f* indicate figures; page numbers followed by *t* indicate tables.

A

ABMTR. *See* Autologous Blood and Marrow Transplant Registry
acupuncture, for pain management, 114
acute promyelocytic leukemia, 72
acyclovir, 84
ADCC. *See* antibody-dependent cellular cytotoxicity
adjuvant agents (coanalgesics), for pain management, 114
Adryamicin (doxorubicin), 68*t*
agarose, 34
Akt, 129
Al amyloidosis, 27
albumin, 34, 40, 51
α globulins, 35–36
α₁ globulins, 35
α₁ lipoprotein (HDL), 35
α₂ globulins, 36
alkylating agents, 67, 68*t*
allogeneic stem cell transplant, 107–110
nonmyeloablative, 108–109
syngeneic, 110

American Cancer Society, 1
American Society of Clinical Oncology, 113
American Society of Hematology, 113
amino acids, 14
amyloid protein, 33
amyloidosis, 34, 38
anemia, 9, 111–113
angiogenesis, 12, 21
inhibitors, 128
anthracycline, 78
anti-CD3 T cells, 76
anti-MAG antibodies, 121
antibodies. *See also* immunoglobulins
panel, 50
monoclonal. *See* monoclonal antibodies
antibody-dependent cellular cytotoxicity (ADCC), 88
antidepressants
for peripheral neuropathy, 121
for pain management, 114
antiepileptics, for peripheral neuropathy, 121

lymphoid cells, 69
    progenitor, 15
lymphoma, 27

M

M-component. *See* monoclonal
    spike (M-spike)
M protein, 14
Macintyre, William, 9
macrophage inflammatory
        protein 1-α (MIP-1α),
        20, 22
magnetic resonance imaging
        (MRI), 43
    spinal, 120
    for thoracic spine, 43*f*
maintenance therapy, 104–106
malignant plasma cells, 8, 45, 45*f*
    transformation, 17
mammalian target of rapamycin
        (mTOR), 129
MAPK pathway. *See* mitogen-
        activated protein kinase
        (MAPK) pathway
Marschalko, Tamas, 10
mass effect, 45
matched unrelated-donor (MUD)
        transplant, 107
Mayo Stratification of Myeloma
        and Risk-Adapted
        Therapy (mSMART), 54*t*
Mcl-1, 130
MDR. *See* multiple drug
        resistance
melphalan, 11, 68*t*, 69, 73, 91, 93,
        96, 98
memory cell, 16

mesenchymal cells, 23
messenger RNA (mRNA), 131
meta-analysis, 71
MFC. *See* multi-parametric flow
        cytometry
MGUS. *See* monoclonal
        gammopathy of
        undetermined
        significance
microarray analysis, 48–49
microvascular density (MVD), 21
mini-allogeneic transplant, 109
minimal residual disease (MRD),
        49, 50
    multi-parametric flow
        cytometry, 49–50
    next-generation
        sequencing, 50
MIP-1α. *See* macrophage
        inflammatory protein
        1-α (MIP-1α)
mitochondrial damage, 73
mitogen-activated protein
        kinase (MAPK)
        pathway, 129
MM. *See* multiple myeloma
MMRF. *See* Multiple Myeloma
        Research Foundation
monoclonal antibodies, 14
    daratumumab, 89–90
    elotuzumab, 88–89
monoclonal gammopathy
        of undetermined
        significance (MGUS), 1, 7,
        18, 29*t*, 121
monoclonal spike (M-spike),
        26, 58
Mozobil (plerixafor), 95

O

P